Arthritis and Other Pain Syndromes

What the Others Are Missing

By

Anthony N. Pannozzo, M.D. and Paul A. Pannozzo, M. D.

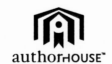

authorHOUSE™

1663 LIBERTY DRIVE, SUITE 200
BLOOMINGTON, INDIANA 47403
(800) 839-8640
WWW.AUTHORHOUSE.COM

© 2004 Anthony N. Pannozzo, M.D. and Paul A. Pannozzo, M.D.
All Rights Reserved.

First published by AuthorHouse 12/08/04

ISBN: 1-4184-9664-2 (sc)
ISBN: 1-4184-9665-0 (dj)

Library of Congress Control Number: 2004096839

Printed in the United States of America
Bloomington, Indiana

This book is printed on acid-free paper.

Disclaimer

The concept of this book is to provide information on pain—its sources and treatment in the perspective of a patient and physician, of which I have both roles. The book is intended to channel your thinking into the best choices you can make for yourself concerning your pain problem. We do not intend to treat you, as you are not a patient of ours and an examination has not taken place. However by all means use the ideas for yourself. I have tried to empower you with knowledge that will help you assess your painful condition to make the right decision for yourself. This book is to educate but not manage your pain complaint.

Each and every effort was made to make this text as complete and accurate as I could. We cannot assume your take on what you are reading, because we cannot write about each and every situation.

Acknowledgements

I am eternally grateful for the opportunity to attend medical school and train at the department of Physical Medicine at the Ohio State University Medical Center. My inspiration is Ernest W. Johnson, M.D., professor and chairman who instilled the concept of proving the diagnosis before treating, trained me in electrodiagnostic testing, and was a dynamic influence over the years. For introducing the concept of facetal injection to me I would like to thank Dr. Maigne. I would like to thank the professors who were responsible for the courses I took in osteopathic treatments, chiropractic manipulation, physical therapy, acupuncture, and scores of other topics, who allowed me to take the best aspects of each to instill them into my daily practice, the results of which are in this book.

My son and colleague Dr. Paul A. Pannozzo has been of inestimable help in writing this book in rounding out research for each topic and developing some of the manuscript. He brings the enthusiasm of the new specialist grounded in the current medical thought from his training in the PM&R department of the Ohio State University Hospitals. We have discussed the topics in this book and proved the concepts and techniques from the academic to actual practice to satisfy the diversity of opinion from the academic and the practical world that we practice in. All of the concepts and procedures have been proven on actual patients.

Table of Contents

Preface

The purpose in writing this book was to fill a void that I noticed in the texts that I was able to read authored by others. I have a unique experience and point of view of musculoskeletal pain honed over 36 years and 45,000 patients. When I started treating musculoskeletal pain all those years ago, the standard for my specialty was to work in an institution directing a large staff, with little direct patient involvement. The experience of treating patients directly has been outstanding for me in a professional and personal sense. The advice given in this text is similar to what you would have heard if I had treated you directly. Of course, I have to disclaim any direct results to you if you read this text, because I have not examined you. The ideas are sound, and proven over those many years and great number of patients. The outcome studies verify the validity of the approaches to pain that are written in this text. The examples given as part of the discussion in the text are from my records. There are thousands of examples not included. Not every pain situation is discussed in these pages. Perhaps some lengthening of some of the chapters will occur later. I have attempted to modify some of the concepts and terms used generally to a different point of view that I feel as a physician and consumer are more accurate, thus empowering you the reader. You are still the one making the decision about your health care. I only hope that some mistakes are now not going to occur. The other practitioners of pain treatment may not always agree with what I have written, however, their comments are welcome. They will be responded to in the future. There are separate chapters written for each pain problem area that I could think about. Obviously I could not comment on all pain problems. You the reader can access our web site to communicate directly if you so choose (www.paintreatment.cc) This is not a referenced text, as you would expect in a book written for physicians. However if we can save one surgery or one headache being treated for long periods without result, then we have achieved the purpose for writing this book.

Introduction

Every family in the world is affected by a member of that family in pain. In the U.S. it is estimated that between 37-45 million people have been affected by a painful condition, and approximately 90% of Americans will have an episode of lower back pain at one time in their lives. The fact that pain is universal to humanity must mean that our bodies cannot handle excessive physical stress because of our construction. I will broaden this concept later. It also means we are doing a poor job of diagnosing and treating causes of pain— more on this later also. This is the reason that there are so many people affected by pain on a long term basis resulting in physical disability, workers compensation disability, and dependence on the welfare system. Over-testing for pain problems and over-treating these syndromes has helped to increase healthcare costs and burden state budgets. This does not even consider the other costs to families, who must shoulder this expense and accommodate the associated emotional difficulties, which cannot be estimated in dollar amounts.

There are various names attached to painful conditions such as migraine, arthritis, slipped disc, herniated disc, bulging disc, degenerative disc disease, and degenerative joint disease. Some names are specific, but most are not. A common diagnosis is lumbar sprain/strain, which does not lend itself to treatment because there is no location given for the diagnosis. This is the first point I can make: If the physician cannot provide a specific diagnosis at a specific location, you cannot be given a specific treatment. That is you will be treated in generalities to an entire region, "treating" structures that do not need to be treated and prolonging your treatment regimen at an increased cost. The diagnosis of failed back syndrome is also a favorite. This diagnosis is given to post-operative spine patients who do not improve from the surgery. No where in this diagnosis does it say that the surgeon misdiagnosed the patient—though it should. Rather, it connotes the back has failed and the patient has failed, almost shifting the onus of responsibility away from the physician, who should know better, to the patient, who does not. There are other non-diagnoses such as fibromyalgia, cephalgia, trigger points, and others. I will explain all of them to you in the appropriate chapter.

There are 20-25 specialty practitioners treating pain, from allopathic physicians to massagers, chiropractors, psychologists, and surgeons. We should not exclude the drug companies, which sell and promote narcotics and other mind-altering drugs, none of which are specific to the origins of the painful conditions. This fact indicates that the causes of pain are not known by most practitioners out there. No practitioner will tell you that their program is guaranteed to reduce pain. Chiropractors and physical therapists cannot predict improvement of pain syndromes in spite of numerous studies and publications. The reason, as noted before, is that they do not have a specific diagnosis, and they follow a failed ideology. None of the methods thus far promoted by these groups have made a significant impact in reducing pain and disabilities.

This industry generates billions of dollars for the practitioners but does not lessen pain. Why are so many people on disability? Why is the United States spending millions on research? We allopathic physicians have failed the mandate and trust of our patients to help them. We have further eroded the science of pain diagnosis and treatment by fostering these other groups because we are not teaching the diagnosis and treatment of musculoskeletal problems in our medical schools and residency programs. Primary care practitioners, ever busy and under a literal mountain of paperwork, simply cannot deal with all these problems effectively. Patients are referred off without specific diagnoses and essentially pushed to physical therapists to do as they wish. Anyone who has held a prescription that stated "Evaluate and Treat" has been in this position. In some states physical therapy has become such an integrated step in the process that patients do not need a prescription to walk in and begin a program. That means a non-physician is making a diagnosis, playing the physician role without the physician knowledge base. We medical doctors have failed the mandate and trust of our patients to help them. In my estimation the poor musculoskeletal education is also directly responsible for the ascendancy of the chiropractor, homeopathic doctor, and other non-allopathic health care providers as disenchanted patients simply seek some kind of answer for their symptoms. We have eroded the science of pain diagnosis and treatment by fostering these other groups, because we are not teaching the diagnosis and proper treatment of musculoskeletal problems in our medical schools and residency programs.

Our economy has suffered markedly because of the non-productive members of society requiring cash payments for being painful. This book is intended to help the public learn what symptoms mean, so proper treatment can be obtained to prevent long term pain. All pain is generated by an incident, such as a fall, lifting, sports, tripping, or other trauma. We are not born painful. Aging in itself cannot produce a disabling pain—there is no gene for producing pain. In this book I will try to educate you on my approach for understanding and treating these pain syndromes, which has been developed over 35 years and 45,000 patients. The explanations you will read here are given to my private patients. We are not attempting to treat the readers of this book, because it is impossible to do so without a history, physical exam, and special films that I do routinely.

As I started to see more patients I realized that the approaches that were common to my training were not as productive as I wanted them to be. I was looking for a complete diagnosis and faster treatments, and I began to question the principles that I was taught. The concept of the engineering of the spine to bear weight was similar to the physics of weight bearing in the physical environment. Design and function of the spine and other joints conceptually took place over the years with gradual evolution to the current anatomy. How was the construction of the lumbar spine designed to not only bear weight, but to do it in motion? What design permitted the knee and hip to be so able to bear weight in smaller and larger people? Why does a foot carry a 100 pound person and a 350 pound person? The bone structure is essentially the same in everyone. The physiology of the spine was my first endeavor to understand the structure of normal as opposed to the abnormal or painful function. I went back to the text books and reread everything I had learned with the thought of design and function from a physics perspective. The results are in this book, tailored to the general public. Later I intend to produce a text for the teaching of these principles to health care providers.

I have had an interest in acute pain diagnosis and treatment from my earliest time in training to the present day. My friend and teacher Ernest W. Johnson, M.D. gave me a chance to study musculoskeletal medicine at the Ohio State University School of Medicine, Physical Medicine Department, in 1964, where the emphasis was on electrodiagnostic studies for nerve and muscles diseases. I came to realize that testing was not the final use of my training, but rather to evaluate and alleviate pain.

The last 35 years, 45,000 patients, millions of treatments, and thousands of injections have brought down the number of days required to treat pain problems. As my skills in diagnosis improved, proven by the treatments which followed, certain hypotheses became truths. These truths explained the mechanism of pain production, which I am calling *the failure to bear weight*, or *the failure of the normal physiology of weight bearing*. These concepts will be explained clearly and in simple terms in each appropriate chapter. I was able to treat a low back problem early on in 6 weeks, later reducing it to 3 weeks, and now most of the problems are treated overnight. It is shocking but true. Where there are many sources of pain, it usually takes one to two days to treat each source. These results are predictable and reproducible, which are the hallmarks of understanding, thus a science.

This book is written with the perspective of a physician and also a patient. I have had most of the syndromes that will be described here. Most of the approaches I use are based on principles I have used for my own treatment. This is quality control at the highest. The ideas put forth in this book have been proven in my own private practice to be valid and have passed the scientific test with predictable results and reproducibility by other doctors using my principles.

The principles of rehabilitation mean that a person with pain will need to attain a normal range of motion without pain, and that is the goal. The experience we have conducting our own treatments without anyone else involved, and sometimes me doing the treatments myself, brings out certain ideas that are not available to physicians who refer patients out to physical therapists, chiropractors, or surgeons to treat. The ideas presented here are to help you cope with the pain that you have by having a better idea of what that pain means, why that pain is produced, and where it is produced. This gives you a better idea when to seek medical care and when not to. The following pages will illustrate these ideas for you to use for your own benefit and pain free state. We are not asking you to be patients of ours but to utilize these ideas to prevent pain and disability, loss of jobs, surgery, and unnecessary treatments.

It is said that the old model of pain is no longer tenable. The old cause and effect idea has given way in some literature to the "new" model of pain that separates the cause of pain to self-generating pain by the body itself. When I read this literature, I cannot help but think that these authors must be talking to themselves and not treating patients. Indeed, a vast part of the literature is written by Ph.D. types who do not have clinical experience and have not had the joy of curing a pain in a real person. When I read this literature, I am struck by the fact that very little is said about where the pain originates. Some of these authors are anesthesiologists not trained in musculoskeletal medicine. These physicians will block a nerve to *make* a diagnosis. I make diagnoses based on the physical examination. These physicians will say that an examination cannot discriminate specific structures to be painful. I know they examine patients with a conceptual basis that I have rejected years ago. Blocking nerves without a proper examination, or doing epidurals without a proper examination, can only lead to this present disaster of thought. Most of these authors do not have a clinical practice, but depend wholly on physical therapists to diagnose and treat patients. When the treatment fails, then the old theory of pain production must be "wrong." This is nowhere near the truth. In these pages, everything I have written has been verified by the old methods of scientific medicine, such as a good history and physical examination as a baseline for treatment and to use this baseline to judge improvement. Only in the pain literature is normal thought thrown out. Does a cardiologist assume that the heart will keep attacking its owner without reason, or do they try to find a cause and effect relationship to find out how to save lives and prevent disability? There can not be a spontaneous firing of nerves. The design and function of the organ will not allow this to happen. It is also said that pain by itself can cause the nervous system and brain to be altered permanently. If the stimulus from the pain source is removed, does this happen?

Every page in this book describes a pain source in terms that can be reasonably reproduced in your doctor's office. This is clinical medicine at its best. You will be able to compare this text with what is told to you by alternative medicine physicians, who may have very little clinical experience with pain.

How is one to take control of his pain if the body spontaneously fires off pain impulses without cause? What good does diet do for this, when foods cannot cause spontaneous firing of nerves? When you think of pain, there is always a source, and therefore it is always diagnosable.

I have had experience in treating phantom limb pain. A patient came to me with the full gamut of symptoms of phantom limb syndrome including so called neuropathic pain and tingling from a below knee amputation. I examined the hip and knee joint as part of the pain pattern. There was a flexion contracture of the knee, secondary to the construction of the prosthesis. But on palpation of the amputation site, I discovered a small swollen area of inflammatory tissue. Palpation of this node produced extreme pain. I injected a steroid into that area, and in 10 minutes, the pain was abating, and the phantom limb sensation was disappearing. This pain and phantom sensation did not return. I checked with the patient on this. The proponents of uncontrollable firing of nerves are wrong on this issue. The nerve connection to the brain is still intact from the limb, and stimulus of this area will get a typical response. If your arm is painful, you certainly can identify the location of that pain, because the nerve system is still intact. Even if that area is treated, the system is still able to re-identify a local source of pain. It appears in the literature that a clinical exam is not done or is done by less skilled personnel. Here is the bottom line on neuropathic pain—it does not exist.

Chapter 1
The Physiology of Pain Production

A pain must be defined in order to understand the origin of that pain. A pain is perceived in the brain as an electrical impulse. Therefore where does that impulse come from? Pain cannot be imagined, because it is the result of a noxious or painful stimulus causing a sensory nerve to fire off, creating an electrical impulse which travels from the source of that pain via the nerve to the spinal cord and then to the sensory areas of the brain. Pain is caused by an injured structure. We know this is true because there is always an antecedent event such as a fall or twisting which caused the symptom—pain does not begin out of the blue. The tissue injury starts an inflammatory change, which is the body's method of repair and begins after any injury. Simply put, injured tissue releases chemicals in the body that promote inflammation, cause nerves to signal pain, and attract repair cells to the injured area. For musculoskeletal pains like back and neck pains, there are only **5** structures in the body to cause a pain other than a fracture or tumor, which are entirely different than the usual causes and will not be considered in this text.

The first structure is a **muscle**. Muscle pain is perceived a day after a strain injury occurs, such as lifting weights in the gym, raking leaves, or lifting the baby, or falling or tripping. In other words, a trauma or accident is the cause. Muscle pain typically lasts for 3-4 days maximally. There is a general soreness where the strain took place, which is in the substance of the muscle tissue. Palpation or squeezing the muscle will produce a typical soreness. There will be no referral of pain to the leg or arm or tingling. Muscle pain will resolve itself in the expected 3-4 days. Aspirin is the best drug for this pain because it is an anti-inflammatory medication. The injury to the muscle may not be clear, but the time for improvement is clear.

The second pain producer is **nerve**. Any nerve has a beginning and an end point. There are two components of any peripheral nerve, which is a nerve away from the spine. These components are the sensory, which allows you to feel, and the motor, which produces movement. If the sensory component is affected there will be a sensory change, like a tingling and mild loss of touch sensation. If the sensory component is severely affected there may be complete numbness in the areas of the body that the nerve serves, which are well known to your physician. If the motor component is affected there will be weakness in the muscles that the nerve goes to. Pure motor nerve diseases, such as polio and amyotrophic lateral sclerosis, or Lou Gehrig's disease, are never painful. Those afflicted have weakness in a specific distribution of the nerve. Another well known example is when someone strikes the back of the elbow hitting the "funny bone", which is actually the ulnar nerve. They will notice a tingling sensation, but it will not be described as a pain usually.

If you have a pain in the leg or the arm without the above sensory or motor changes, it is likely that there is no "pinched nerve", but there are other structures causing that pain. A nerve does not usually cause a pain but when compressed, it will produce a tingling sensation in a specified area that is well known. A typical nerve from the low back such as L_5 will cause tingling to the ankle, top of the foot, and big toe, but very little pain. The surrounding structures causing the nerve to malfunction is actually causing the pain. A nerve should never be touched, or injected, but the surrounding structures must be treated to relieve the pain. The success of treatment is noted very quickly as the tingling is resolved. The principle to understand here is that a pain down the leg is not necessarily a pinched nerve as some will espouse. There are other structures that will cause pain in the arm or leg. Without the tingling and sensory loss in specified areas, there is probably no nerve damage. Peripheral nerves do heal after injury, albeit slowly over time. The cause and severity of any nerve abnormality must be taken into consideration, for many nerve diseases have irreversible changes. Prognosis for each condition should really be discussed with your physician. These abnormalities will be discussed further in this book in other chapters.

The third structure is the **ligament,** which joins bones together. Also included in this category are joint capsules, which surround every joint in the body and connects the bones to each other across the joint. Examples are the hip, knee, shoulder, ankle, and spinal joint capsules. The genius of the design is that the ligament permits the normal motion of the joint, but will not permit motion outside of what we call the normal range of motion. When a trauma or accident takes place, the physical stress on the ligament will cause small pull injuries where it connects to the bone. The ligament attaches to the outer lining of the bone, called the periosteum, where the nerves for the bone are located. These injuries cause an inflammatory change at the periosteum level, causing pain and tenderness. Pain from a joint, or facet joint in the spine, is actually from the capsule, or specifically where the capsule-bone connection takes place. All arthritis is actually a ligament injury. Ligament pain can be quite severe and can last for weeks and months after the injury. It may not resolve until medical treatment is obtained. Your body is not falling apart as some would tell you. There is no pain when flexing a muscle usually. This type of pain is found by examining the passive range of motion.

Ligaments in our body have a typical response to injury. A ligament will be stiffer after inactivity such as sleeping. It will feel somewhat better with increased body temperature, like when lying in the hot tub, and with overstretch, such as when manipulation occurs, but this improvement is only temporary. It will cause pain on stretch. It easily scars down and becomes calcified over time—you see it as spur formation, or repair process of the body. Taking the over stretch away from a painful ligament will heal it rather quickly, that is in days. Injecting it will not cure it unless the cause of the overstretch is treated.

The annulus, or spinal disc, is a ligament as well, joining one vertebral body to the one above and below. The annulus permits rotation and extension and thus is easily examined. An injury to that annulus, which is at the ligament-bone connection, causes an inflammatory change and severe pain which is diagnosed by bending backward, known as extension, and the typical symptomatic pain pattern which will be unique for each annulus. For instance, the annulus between the L_4 and the L_5 vertebral bodies refers to the outside of the calf in the lower leg and down the side of the thigh. Every injured ligament has a specific pain pattern associated with it. Annular pain can persist indefinitely until it is treated properly.

It may be of interest to the reader that the size of the annulus that can cause pain may be less than one inch in length and one-half inch in height, but it can be severe and incapacitating pain. The main point here is that if you can bend backwards without pain in the lower back there is no disc to treat. Likewise the cervical disc problems will not permit looking up, but looking down or chin-to-chest is able to be done. When there is a pain in the neck, or between the shoulder blades, or in the lower back and you are able to bend backwards there is no disc pain. I think of the annulus as a structure of mobility. When that mobility is lost from an injury, then pain will be produced with movement.

The fourth pain producing structure is the **muscle-bone connector**. In some muscles, the main muscle mass attaches directly to the bone without forming a tendon. An example of this type of muscle is the adductor group along the inner thigh. You can feel this muscle on the inside of the thigh. The adductors bring your knees together and your legs forward with walking. In any case the pain producing structure is where the muscle and bone join. The muscle will attach to the outer layer of bone, the periosteum, where the nerves for the bone are located. An injury at this site causes an inflammatory change with pain and is called an enthesitis. A typical example is a muscle cramp, also a "hamstring injury." More severe forms of this injury type can cause a tingling sensation but this is in a more general area than what a nerve would cause. However there will be pain with motion, and sometimes the source of this can be hard to find. See picture below of the adductor muscle to see a broad muscle attachment without a tendon.

The fifth structure is the **tendon-bone connector**. In some muscles, the attachment to the bone is by a tendon, which transmits the contraction of that muscle to the bone. An example of this is the quadriceps muscle, which has a tendon around the patella, or knee cap. The tendon attaches to the periosteum, where the nerves for the bone are located. An injury at this site causes an inflammatory change with pain and is called a tendonitis. There will be pain and tenderness at the site where the tendon inserts into the bone. There will be pain on contraction of the muscle. See picture below.

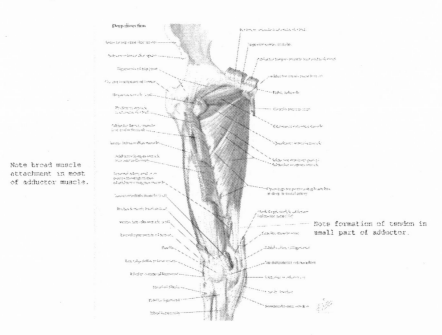

Common to all of these injured structures is inflammation at the injury site. The body will repair any injury through the process of inflammation by producing scar tissue at that area as a repair process. The body is simply trying to heal and protect itself by making a strong scar, to give that tissue strength so further injury does not occur. The scar tends to attract calcium and this scar tissue may become hard and bone-like over time. This is sometimes described as spur formation on x-ray and usually called "arthritis". The term arthritis should not be used for this process because it is merely the result of the process of repair. Another example of this is a bone spur commonly found on the heel bone. The plantar fascia had been pulled from its attachment to the bone, and the scar tissue produced though repair has been calcified.

The goal for treatment therefore is to decrease the inflammatory change that is occurring, consequently decreasing the pain and increasing the range of motion. All pain is derived from the described structures, either singly or in combination, with inflammation always involved. This concept eliminates several treatment approaches to pain problems, like narcotics, muscle relaxants, and any other mind-altering drugs which are not anti-inflammatory, manipulation, or exercise during pain. It also eliminates the concept of weakness causing pain.

The diagnosis and treatment of the pain producing structures is a combination of the above. Sometimes the annulus and joint are injured at the same time. The treatment of both of these structures can be done simultaneously. When I examine a patient for pain syndromes, the part being examined, such as the neck, lower back, shoulder, or hip, the normal physiology, or design and function, of that structure goes through my mind. The location of the structure is recorded and then an x-ray film is used to develop the approach to treat it. Many times an abnormal structure cannot be seen on x-ray or MRI. The reason for this is that the painful structures are normal but are interacting abnormally.

How does an injury occur? To understand how an injury occurs we must first talk about form and function. For example a sphere is designed to roll but a cube is designed for weight bearing. The spine was designed to bear weight as we stand upright and also in motion using three points in a triangular formation—the annular ligament at the front corner between the vertebral bodies and a facet joint on each posterior corner. This can be easily seen in the picture below as an outlined triangle superimposed on the picture:

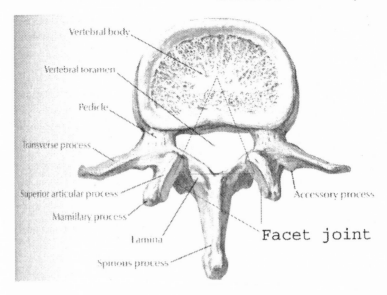

The vertebral bodies are connected to each other by ligaments that allow motion, giving the spine a normal ability to bear weight and allow pain free motion, which we call the normal physiology of weight bearing. When we discuss physiology we mean the smooth workings of the muscles and ligaments and nerves in the way they were designed. For example, in order for the neck to do the marvelous movements that we all know, several things must take place simultaneously. There is a complex coordinated set of motions using the bone structures, muscles, and ligaments, which must be flexible enough to allow mobility. The structures described above can only perform the way they were designed to do so. Therefore the smooth two-sided motion of the normal spine is the normal physiology of weight bearing. Flexion, extension, and rotation are only possible if all three components are freely moveable on all sides. Any restriction, then, will cause a deviation of the spinal column wherever that restriction takes place. This has nothing to do with muscle or nerves but has everything to do with ligament structure.

Pain therefore is an abnormal physiology and is a manifestation of an injured structure. A pain source causes a reduced, painful motion. In other words, a pain can be defined for this examination as *the inability to stretch*. The ligament causing pain will not be able to stretch. This is what we call the failed physiology of weight bearing.

7

This makes sense because motion is normal, no motion, or painful motion is abnormal, and this is treated so the motion returns to a pain free state, which is freely moveable, or as we say a "normal range of motion." The idea is that the medical examination is designed to find that structure and treat it appropriately. The location of that pain, and the reason for that, is where the clinician must understand the intricate detail of how the spine works. Misunderstanding of these principles is the basis for chronic pain. This concept can be generalized to the hips, knees, ankles, shoulders, and all other joints of the body.

See picture:

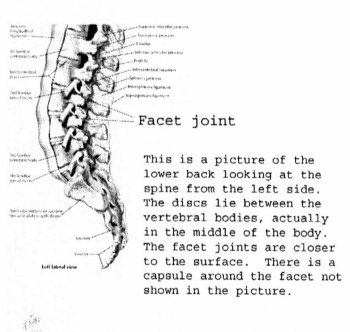

Facet joint

This is a picture of the lower back looking at the spine from the left side. The discs lie between the vertebral bodies, actually in the middle of the body. The facet joints are closer to the surface. There is a capsule around the facet not shown in the picture.

There is another fact to remember when discussing the normal physiology of weight bearing: there are two facets working together. This must never be forgotten. If a joint on one side were to have restricted motion there will be a hyper mobile joint movement on the opposite side. This is because of the "swivel effect"—the spine will swivel on the injured, restricted side, causing the mobile joint to assume more of the motion of that segment. And as we mentioned above, a ligament structure allows a limited range of motion, and any movement beyond this defined range will be painful. Conversely, pain can originate from the scarred side as well. The clinician must be well versed in this understanding to discriminate the actual pain generator. Extending these basic principles leads us to determine that a flexion, or forward leaning pain, is from the facet joints, while a pain with extension, or bending backward, originates from the annulus. This scenario has been tested and retested over 45,000 patients and is absolutely true.

Of the major joints in the body that produce pain, the actual pain producing structure is the joint capsule, which surrounds every joint and is itself a ligament. As stated earlier, the ligament allows normal motion and inhibits abnormal motion, thereby allowing a "normal range of motion." Joint capsules can be injured on one side, thus causing the "swivel effect". One side of the joint capsule will allow decreased motion, and the opposite side will consequently have increased relative motion. When the ligament structure of the major joints exceeds the allowable motion designed in the joint, an injury occurs and, therefore, a pain occurs. It is up to the physician to examine properly to find the ultimate cause of the pain. This is the same process in all of the joints, including shoulders, hips, knees, ankles, elbows, and wrists. All these concepts will be described in detail in later chapters.

Glossary

Annulus: In general, a synonym for intervertebral disc. The disc is comprised of the annulus and the nucleus pulposis.

Inflammation: The body's method of repair. This process begins after any injury, from a simple scrape to an ankle sprain to a bullet wound. Injured tissue causes chemicals to be released which cause nerves to signal pain, increase blood flow to the area, and attract white blood cells to repair the area and begin scar formation.

Facet Joint: Joint between two vertebral arches which dictates the range of motion of the area of the spine because of its location and construction. The facet joints are paired and located just beneath the muscles of the back at the bone.

9

Ligament: Any tissue connector between two bones.

Musculoskeletal: Relating to muscle and bones.

Palpation: To examine by touch.

Physiology: A branch of biology that deals with the functions and activities of life or of living matter (as organs, tissues, or cells) and of the physical and chemical phenomena involved.

Sprain: Ligament injury.

Strain: Muscle injury.

Subluxation: A spinal vertebral joint, sliding into the lower joint.

Swivel Effect: A phenomenon that is related to the two sided motion of all joints.

Tendon: A specialized part of the muscle that joins the fleshy muscle belly to the bone.

Chapter 2
Testing, Terminology, and Misconceptions

Testing
<u>Testing</u>

With musculoskeletal pain syndromes, there are many tests available however only a few that we feel are of any value. The tests can be thought of as "physiologic" or "anatomic". Physiologic studies require a patient to be alive and breathing for any result. They are dynamic tests that reflect how the body is functioning at that moment in time and require the patient and tester to be there at the same time. Examples of these are the bone scan, electromyogram and nerve conduction studies, standing X-Ray and others. The electrocardiogram, for heart patients, would also be a test of this kind. The discogram is also a physiologic test, however it is inaccurate and too painful for me to consider useful. I will describe these tests in more detail later below.

The standing anterior-posterior, or front-to-back, **spine x-ray** film is useful because it is a weight-bearing film and shows us how the individual bears weight in the normal position. We take our lower back films so that it includes the pelvis and hip joints. The film reflects the way people are at that moment in time, and also what injuries they have incurred in the past. This test shows the side-to-side view of the individual bearing weight through the spine in the normal fashion. We are also able to determine if there is a leg-length inequality and then show our correction in a scientific manner. The radiograph identifies any curvatures or pelvic obliquity and is used after the clinical exam determines which structure is causing pain. This film is used to develop a treatment program based on the clinical diagnosis. For example, if on clinical exam there is a pain on bending on the right side and we determine it is between the third and the fourth vertebra, we then look at the standing film to see what is affecting that particular structure. A treatment program is then designed for the findings at that particular time. In no way is the film used to diagnose the source of pain. Pain is diagnosed on a clinical basis only, because it is the culmination of several physiologic processes, and the patient needs to be involved in locating the pain and when it occurs during the examination.

The **electromyogram**, or EMG, is an objective type test that cannot be changed by the patient or examiner. It is done with an exploring needle electrode that is inserted into a muscle. It is extremely valuable because it is a physiologic test and reflects the past and current health of the nerve studied. It should be performed on any patient prior to a surgical procedure for pain relief. We believe that EMGs should also be performed before any epidural injection. The herniated disc, which is supposedly highly inflammatory to the nerve root, should cause changes in the nerve if that were the cause for pain. All too frequently however, physicians perform epidural injections without this test, and the results may not be favorable to the patient. These physicians are usually anesthesiologists who do not share the neuro-musculoskeletal background that physiatrists have. Recently at a physician conference I was discussing this issue with an anesthesiologist who did not know why I would order an EMG for a radiculopathy-type pain complaint. He thought I wanted to investigate lumbar muscle spasms. This really made we wonder how ineffective and inefficient the typical pain physician is in their work.

EMGs should be ordered if any kind of true nerve or muscle weakness is suspected from the history or found on the physical examination, for example a foot drop. This test helps to determine if the weakness is due to pain, which causes muscle inhibition, or actual nerve or muscle disease. The EMG should never be skipped in any workup of the patient with the appropriate clinical picture.

The **bone scan** is also an excellent physiologic test. A radioactive solution is injected into the bloodstream and in two hours it is absorbed at areas of inflammation. A camera takes a picture of the body and is able to show where this solution was absorbed. We know that pain is secondary to an inflammatory change; therefore this test can be quite helpful. It is also able to detect other causes of pain, for example cancer. The localization of the solution to the structure makes it a useful test.

The other tests available are anatomic studies, which are less useful. These tests are static and do not even require the patient to be alive for a result. They provide anatomical relationships only, and are incapable of localizing any source of pain. Examples of these are supine X-Ray, MRI, CT scan (cat scan), myelogram, and others. These tests cannot tell you where a pain is originating from with any amount of accuracy. To make my point, I own an atlas that has pictures of normal MRI anatomy for necks and backs and brains. This atlas was made from MRI examinations performed on cadavers. That MRI image proves nothing beyond basic anatomy. For another example, 30% of people with no back pain will have "herniated discs" on a lumbar MRI. This is an anatomic abnormality to be sure, however not a physiologic cause of pain in these instances. If the MRI was performed in the standing position, for example, it would increase its accuracy though would still need proper interpretation.

As a consumer of health care as you and I are, I would be extremely concerned about having an MRI that shows a herniated disc or any other abnormality that is not accompanied by a restricted range of motion of that area. Most of the time these are isolated findings and do not correlate well with the clinical exam. What we usually see from our dynamic standing X-Ray is *why* that abnormality is there on the MRI.

Terminology and Misconceptions

There are many terms that are bandied about around the country and in the medical literature. Many are aimed toward you, the consuming public. I am a member of the consuming public and I will attempt to put these words into perspective for you.

13

<u>Spinal Instability</u>

It is said in the literature of physical therapists and physicians that spine pain originates through a failure of one of three proposed influences on the spine. These three subsystems are the (1) static stabilizers, or ligaments, (2) dynamic structures, or muscles, and (3) neural elements, like the nerves and spinal cord. This theory has not been proven, and in my estimation, it will never be. The reason is the 5 structures we have discussed previously have not been mentioned as primary pain generators in this theory and there is no mention of any actual injury, just a "failure" of one of the three subsystems. What is a "failure"? How does this "failure" occur? What is the actual cause of pain? How does this "failure" lead to overall "dysfunction"? As you can see, there is no depth and no scientific understanding in this theory in my opinion. I do not use this concept for my patients or myself or my family members.

The error is in their idea that pain comes from weakness in muscular forces, which allows too much motion in the spine, thereby putting an imbalance on joints and ligaments. These structures are thought to be unable to take the stress and therefore become painful. The fallacy here is that people with acute injuries get them while twisting, lifting, or other catastrophic events. They exceed the physiologic ability to bear weight in motion as we described above. The hypermobility, if any, is secondary to joint or ligament structure primarily, as a "swivel effect" which we will explain in detail in later chapters. The muscle is doing the only job it can do, which is contract. The people are not weak, but painful. One can also ask why the individual was pain free the day before the inciting event which caused the pain, though the back must have had the same strength before the event and after. As anyone knows strength is stable with use—muscles do not weaken unless not used. When the pain source is treated successfully and quickly, there is no evidence of weakness at all.

The treatment method espoused through this theory is to find a "neutral position" where your pain is least and to try to maintain that position as much as possible. These treatment programs can last for weeks and usually do not provide significant help. I feel that motion should be *encouraged,* and a normal range of motion should be attained by localizing and treating the painful structure.

This is a good example of people, without a clinical practice such as I have, coming to conclusions that are unexplainable. As I have stated before, mobility is the key, not strength. I would advise anyone carrying a diagnosis of "spinal instability" to go elsewhere. Remember the five sources of pain—each one needs to be evaluated and treated separately.

Muscle Pain and Spasm

Back pain is usually attributed to muscle strain and "spasms". This is in reference to the muscle belly, or muscle tissue. Often the muscles around the spine can be felt to be tight and contracted. The muscle will be sore to the touch. Patients may often be provided muscle relaxers or given trigger point injections to treat this supposed problem. A muscle can certainly be painful—we have all had muscle pulls, for example the hamstring, when there is true injury to the contractile elements. However injuries to the muscle belly tend to heal over two to three days because of a very good blood supply.

Muscle belly pain needs to be separated from muscular insertion pain and ligament pain. Symptoms can be similar and at times the locations of each type of structure may be essentially the same. People with muscle strain injuries will still have a normal range of motion of that joint. In contrast ligament injuries prevent a normal range of motion and tend to last longer. Muscle insertion pain is worsened with active contraction of the muscle and will have tenderness at the site where it meets the bone. A certain level of anatomic knowledge is essential for this localization. This critical distinction is made because they are treated differently. Muscle insertion pain is treated locally. Ligament is mobilized to allow a normal range of motion. We do not believe in muscle relaxers or trigger point injections because muscle belly pain is not the cause of any long-term pain. A few days of anti-inflammatories are usually sufficient. The concept of "spasm" or uncontrolled muscle contraction is erroneous. It actually is a guarding action of the body to prevent movement of a painful bone structure below it.

Chronic Pain

The term *chronic pain*, in my opinion, should never be used because it only refers to how long an individual has had the pain, not from where the pain originates. No pain is continuous for six months as the term would suggest. Pain of any kind is intermittent in nature over time, worse some days than others. Therefore this more fits the concept of episodic acute injury and therefore able to be treated. This is important because the concept of chronic pain, if followed, connotes that an individual is undiagnosable and incurable, therefore the treatment of choice is narcotics, mind altering drugs, disability, and an overload of procedures. There are a limited number of structures that will cause pain. Psychology and emotion have nothing to do with pain sources, but how each patient interprets his symptoms. The doctor should allay these fears and not promote dire consequences.

Degenerative Joint Disease/Osteoarthritis

The most common painful joint diseases affecting most of us is so called osteoarthritis (OA) or degenerative joint disease (DJD). There are many other joint diseases described but they are usually components of other diseases. OA follows injuries and manifests itself by stiffness, pain, and calcification of ligaments on X-Ray. It is commonly referred to the "wear and tear" changes on the joint. This is not to be thought of as arthritis but rather as a repair process of the body.

As we described above all injuries are based on an inflammatory process and should be treated with anti-inflammatories. It has been stated in the literature that osteoarthritis is actually a non-inflammatory condition. New information is changing that assumption. The joint capsule has been found to have high levels of inflammatory chemicals that cause destruction of the normal capsular tissue. This leads to stiffness and immobility of the capsule because this injured tissue cannot stretch to allow motion like it normally should.

Examination of end-stage joints will not show the inflammatory process—it happened years before. The abnormal calcification reflects this past inflammation and repair. We know that calcium deposition follows tissue injury. When the body attempts to heal

16

and protect itself, it tries to make the tissue stronger. Calcium is laid down in the tissue, which gives it bony toughness. This deposition of calcium about the joint is referred to as "joint hypertrophy" or as "osteophytes" but the underlying reason is similar in nearly all cases. The faster an injury is treated the less calcium formation occurs over time.

Degenerative Disc Disease

This is described to be the "breakdown" or degeneration of the spinal discs. In actuality what this means is a previous injury, inflammation, and repair. The loss of disc height, dehydration, fragility of the disc material, and other findings should be considered as a result of the injury and repair process. There is no instance of "degeneration" as such, and is a misnomer and should not be used. There is as yet no recognized gene that produces a degenerative condition. This wording connotes an unexplainable and unstoppable process without cause, which must be endured. This conclusion is not based on the facts as I have presented them is this book. All the spinal discs are the same age, yet some are more affected than others. This fact alone must show that there are other forces driving this condition.

If you look at lumbar MRIs, you would see the difference between a normal disc and a "degenerated" one. The normal discs have a visible fluid component in the middle and retained height, while the abnormal disc will be darker and flatter. It is not uncommon to see a lumbar MRI with a normal appearing L_5-S_1 disc with markedly "degenerated" discs at the L_{4-5} and L_{3-4} levels. This helps to make the point I am trying to impress. Most motion in the lumbar spine occurs at the L_5-S_1 disc, yet in this example this disc is normal in appearance and the L_{4-5} disc and L_{3-4} disc are abnormal. The degeneration phenomenon cannot be a natural process only related to age. Disc degeneration is caused by an injury which over time causes these changes to accelerate and magnify in severity. This injury can be localized to a specific spinal level where the changes will be the greatest. This is significant because that area can be treated by local treatments and mobilization exercises when properly prescribed. Surgeries are not necessary. The structures to be treated are the annulus and joint capsule. We excel in distinguishing the two and providing a treatment program for each. I have often played a game with the patient to try to age the injury. Most of the time I am on the mark for the time that the injury occurred. Even if the patient does not remember when he was injured, the wife does, or he tells me the date later. This works.

Lumbar sprain/strain or Cervical sprain/strain

Classically the term strain refers to muscle injury and sprain refers to ligament injury. However neither term shows the location of the injury nor reflects on the mechanism of injury. Without knowing these two facts treatment will be less effective. We do not use the term sprain or strain in my practice because it is non-specific. I believe this diagnosis is part of the problem of the worker's compensation system in Ohio and other parts of the country.

The diagnosis of cervical or lumbar sprain is made when a patient presents to their doctor complaining of pain in the neck or back but there are no signs of a radiculopathy or "pinched nerve". The only findings will usually be limitation of range of motion and some tenderness. Physical therapy is ordered, muscle relaxers, anti-inflammatories, and pain pills are prescribed and the patient is re-examined in a few weeks. There is usually no attempt by the physician to make a specific diagnosis and no demand by the state to get a specific diagnosis.

Patients cannot be treated properly when the only diagnosis is a sprain/strain. It is impossible to treat the pain when it is not known what, why, and where. Patients will be better served if the diagnosis is tightened. Those who cannot localize the painful structure should not be recognized as treating pain.

Radiculopathy/ Sciatica/ "Pinched Nerve"

The term "pinched nerve" is used extensively by chiropractors and general practitioners to describe any pain in the lower or upper limb. This does not convey to you the actual source of this pain, however. There are many sources of pain in the leg, the least of which is the pinched nerve or nerve compromise, known as radiculopathy in the medical literature. The other structures we described above can also produce lower extremity pain without nerve involvement.

This fact should put you at ease such that pain in the leg is not always of dire consequences and of a serious nature.

Radiculopathies are thought to be secondary to direct nerve root compression from a disc protrusion or secondary to a chemical process that causes inflammation around the root. This does not give any indication of why this process developed though. Radicular pain, or nerve pain, is specific and follows the path of the nerve, as stated previously. It is described as a tingle or pins-and-needles sensation. An L_5 radiculopathy is most common, and will refer pain to the lateral calf, ankle, and large toe. An S_1 radiculopathy will refer symptoms to the posterior calf and little toe. There are also findings on the examination that point to this diagnosis. When a radiculopathy is present the muscles that get served by that nerve root are weaker because the impulse cannot travel across the inflamed area. There will also be a change in the muscle reflex for that level. As stated before the EMG is the most sensitive test for this diagnosis. Cervical nerve roots can be affected as well, though this is much less common than in the lumbar spine. The C_6 root will refer symptoms to the thumb, the C_7 root will refer to the long finger, and the C_8 will refer to the little finger. These are the three most common cervical radiculopathies.

In addition to the causes of the lower back, the hip can cause pain in the lower limbs and the adductor muscle can cause pain in the lower limb, both of which are commonly overlooked. The knee can cause calf pain, especially while seated, and the night time calf cramps is usually from the back of the knee joint.

If a pain occurs in the lower limb on walking or upon arising from a chair or getting out of bed in the morning, it is actually a hip pain and not a back pain. If the pain arises from the middle of the thigh and down the leg, the pain is muscular in origin and local to that area. If the pain occurs only in the calf, then the source is most likely the knee capsule.

We hear about vascular causes for lower limb pain, however if a pain is to be vascular in origin there must be other associated symptoms. There should be cold, pale feet with delayed capillary refill in the nails if there is an arterial problem. There should be swelling and calf tenderness if there is a veinous problem. If the feet are warm and pink and there is no abnormal swelling, there does not appear to be a vascular cause. There are tests available for vascular insufficiencies, but these other symptoms are needed to justify the testing.

To protect yourself from excessive surgeries, you must be treated by a physician able to isolate the painful area through examination, and then able to begin appropriate treatment. For example, if you are able to isolate a painful area in the mid-thigh or calf, it should be stretched with your hand or treated with an injection if severe enough. Do not accept the term pinched nerve or sciatica as a diagnosis, because they only describe a pain but do not diagnose its origin.

Failed Back Syndrome

The term "Failed Back Syndrome" does not adequately describe what has happened to the patient with multiple surgeries. The term should be thought of as describing the surgeon and not the patient. *Excessive surgeries without a benefit* is what is meant by this term. This can be applied to not only excessive surgeries but also to single fusions of the cervical and lumbar spine. The same principles of 'cause and effect relationships' and 'structures causing pain' have not changed in these patients. The methods we have described above, namely an adequate history and examination to produce a pain and special film to show weight bearing are still true. The only difference is that now there is introduction of scar tissue but its localization and mobilization, and therefore treatment, are still the same. We do not accept the diagnosis of Failed Back Syndrome, as it is a dead-end term. Proper diagnoses are the key to prevent this from happening.

Whiplash

The term whiplash is bandied about quite often after automobile accident. However analysis of the term "whiplash" shows there is no depth to the term and provides no insight to the diagnosis, mechanism of injury, or location of the injury, and it should not be used with any finality.

When we are driving and then hit from behind the neck tends to extend until it is stopped by ligament structure or the headrest. Next the head moves forward, flexing the neck to an extreme degree causing facet joint pain. Side-to-side motions also need to be considered, which change the injury dramatically and occur because of having the head turned at the time of impact. For example, looking to the left at time of impact would hurt the left facet joints more than the right joints. This nullifies the idea that if there is no damage to the car then the person inside could not be injured.

The proper terminology would be to describe a flexion-extension injury if the accident occurred from the front or back, modified by the limitations of the cervical spine previous to the injury and where the person was looking, left or right.

The way you should look at a neck injury is if you can touch your chin to your chest you have no joint problem, and if you can raise your chin you have no disc problem. You can start this examination for yourself by starting with your chin at the resting position, that is straight ahead.

Spinal Stenosis

Spinal stenosis is a radiographic diagnosis made when measurement of the space between the vertebral body and the bony elements in the back is less than a certain distance, 10mm in the lumbar spine for central stenosis and less than 4mm from the facet joint to the vertebral body. This encroachment on the neural elements is usually related to a combination of disc bulge, ligament hypertrophy, and facet joint hypertrophy, which is large calcium build-up on the joints that pushes into the spinal canal. This build-up, as mentioned previously, is related to a remote injury and the body's natural repair process.

This should be thought of as a syndrome and not a diagnosis. I have made a study of the patients that have had this syndrome. The most common finding is a severe subluxation of one lumbar vertebra into another, which causes a narrowing of the spinal canal at that level, and can cause compromised spinal nerve function because of the narrow space on the subluxed side and the stretched area on the opposite side. Subluxation means that one vertebra has slid into another one at the joint level.

Treatment for this is mobilization of the narrowed side to regain the flexibility that was lost. This usually occurs through a severe lifting from one side or a fall on the buttock of the narrowed side.

Usually a flexion exercise, standing with your feet shoulder width apart, and touching the palm of the left hand to the front of the left shin to stretch the right back and touching the palm of the right hand to the front of the right shin to stretch the left back are helpful. We also recommend a left and right side bend to stretch the opposite sides of the back. When the symptoms abate then the need for the exercise is diminished. Aspirin is still the best drug because it is anti-inflammatory, but if the stiffness is more severe a short course of prednisone may be necessary.

Plantar Fasciitis

One of the most disturbing diagnoses in patients with foot pain is so called Plantar Fasciitis. The plantar fascia is a layer of connective tissue that starts at the heel and goes forward to insert along the front part of the arch. This is commonly thought to get stretched and painful from walking. My experience with people who carry this diagnosis is that they get treated many times without benefit. In general, if someone receives many treatments without benefit you can be sure the diagnosis is incorrect.

The usual treatment for plantar fasciitis is to stretch the Achilles muscles and inject the heel where the fascia inserts. Usually people complain that it does not offer relief. Also inserts are sold, which I maintain are of no true benefit. It is said there is a spur at the bottom of the foot which causes an inflammation of the plantar fascia. What you should know as a consumer is that nearly everyone has a spur formation, or calcification of the ligament, on the bottom of the heel seen on X-Ray.

Looking into this problem and doing basic research in my office, it was quite evident the pain of the plantar fasciitis is actually coming from above at the talo-calcaneal ligament, a connector between two bones of the ankle. See picture below.

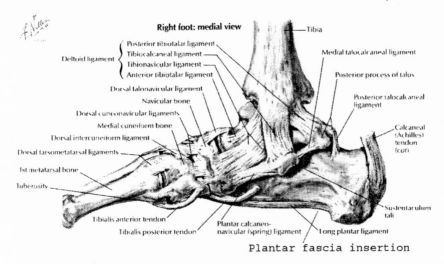

Right foot: medial view

Posterior tibiotalar ligament
Tibiocalcaneal ligament
Deltoid ligament
Tibionavicular ligament
Anterior tibiotalar ligament
Dorsal talonavicular ligament
Navicular bone
Dorsal cuneonavicular ligaments
Medial cuneiform bone
Dorsal intercuneiform ligament
Dorsal tarsometatarsal ligaments
1st metatarsal bone
Tuberosity
Tibialis anterior tendon
Tibialis posterior tendon

Tibia
Medial talocalcaneal ligament
Posterior process of talus
Posterior talocalcaneal ligament
Calcaneal (Achilles) tendon (cut)
Sustentaculum tali
Plantar calcaneo-navicular (spring) ligament
Long plantar ligament

Plantar fascia insertion

The medial talocalcaneal ligament is directly above the area where the plantar fascia inserts, and is directly responsible for heel pain of this type.

We know that because we treat this area with injection using an anesthetic and steroid used to soften the ligament and take the inflammation from the area. In ten minutes that pain is reduced. My technique is to reduce the pain and ask the patient to produce the pain if they can. If we were correct then the pain cannot be produced. We know it is a cure because the people we see a few days later do not have the pain at all, including at the heel bone. It is routine for them to say that prior to treatment the heel was very tender, and they did not even realize they had tenderness where we actually treat. After our treatment, which is not to the heel bone, the heel is not tender to the touch. We find the area that is causing the pain by a meticulous history and physical examination which is unique to our approach.

Neuropathic pain

Neuropathic pain is defined as a nerve "dysfunction", whose etiology is in the central or peripheral nervous system. In simple terms, this refers to pain from nerves themselves without stimulus. They exhibit signs of being abnormal in their own right, firing off signals at random, and causing pain without a reason. It is thought that there are changes in the spinal cord from plasticity of nerve

23

tissue when overly stimulated, causing irreversible changes in that nerve tissue.

My comment to this scenario is to look at it again. There are elements of truth to this theory, but the conclusions are mistaken. Remember there must always be an initial source for the pain. I have treated successfully those who exhibit all of the findings of neuropathic pain by the normal exam that I do every day. The pain sources are found and treated in turn.

Hypersensitized nerves refer to the occasional patient who has so much pain that they cannot stand anyone touching them. Again, the physician should not be overwhelmed by this patient. He is mainly depressed and uncooperative with the examiner, because he suspects that this is another dead end. But a methodical approach to pain sources will allay all fears of this type of patient so the real work of treating him can begin. There is no mechanism of pain production which would cause this type of general response. Remember the term mechanism of disease.

Another facet in the neuropathic pain concept is actual nerve disease, like multiple sclerosis or stroke or any other injury to the brain or spinal cord. Damage to nerves in the brain or spinal cord, known as the central nervous system, leads to what is called the Upper Motor Neuron Syndrome. This differs from what was described above because that referred to a pain stimulus from the periphery causing changes in the central nervous system. The symptoms of the upper motor neuron syndrome include spasticity, which is a change in the muscle that make it is less stretchable and more active. The muscle is also overly sensitive with exaggerated reflex responses to pain. You may have noticed a person who had a stroke hold the arm bent at the elbow and wrist, which is a common example of spastic muscles in the arm and forearm. Multiple Sclerosis will have this symptom, as will spinal cord injury, and severe concussion injury. A spastic muscle is always contracting very strongly and will constantly pull on the bone where it connects. The muscle will actually pull itself out of the bone slightly, causing extreme pain. This pull type injury causes an inflammatory change at the muscle-bone connector.

Physicians are taught to treat spasticity by stretching it in physical therapy or giving a medication to relax the muscle. These anti-spasticity drugs can be taken by mouth or now can be injected directly into the muscle. The prevailing idea is that the muscle belly itself is painful because of the contraction and usually any examiner is taught to look there mostly. At no time in my training did I read or hear anything about examining the origin and insertion of the muscle and treating the pain generator at that site. It is overlooked, but I have found that treating the muscle-bone connector site must be done for the best results. I place a small amount of steroid and pain killer at the connector site and it stops the pain, reduces the uncontrolled reflex muscle contraction, and allows more voluntary motion. I would encourage anyone with spasticity to consider this if their pain has not been treated adequately. The take away idea from this is that often spasticity can be treated on a local basis if the source of irritant can be located at the muscle-bone connector of the leg or arm. I have done research on this over the years.

Migraine

Migraine is a total misnomer. There are whole areas of the medical field and pharmaceutical companies enlisted to treat this problem. The term migraine is to me a one sided pain only, in other words a description and not a diagnosis. The latest opinion is that migraine is from an inflammatory process of the fifth cranial nerve and its nerve body. The only problem with this is that there are twelve cranial nerves, and these people offer no explanation how this inflammatory process strikes only one of the twelve nerves without spreading to other nerves or causing loss of strength in muscles of the fifth nerve. They also do not offer reasons for treating this inflammatory condition with beta-blockers, calcium channel blockers, or anti-seizure medications that offer no anti-inflammatory effects. All headaches come from the inability of the neck to bear weight of the head, which stresses the ligament structure, which causes referred pain which we perceive as headache. The cervical annulus causes dull headache, while the facet joint complex causes the throbbing type headache. I am convinced that the headache described as migraine can be treated successfully as we have done in the past. I do not know if the so called headache clinics cure this problem. I doubt it. There is more discussion of this topic in Chapter 5.

Anthony N. Pannozzo, M.D. and Paul A. Pannozzo, M.D.

A Final Word

As a consumer and patient as you and I are, we need a medical dictionary handy to be educated when medical terms are used. I remember a particular patient who was being seen by a chiropractor, who had given him about 10 diagnoses. They were mainly made up words to describe the location of a pain, such as Cephalgia, which is head pain, and Sciatica, which is leg pain. The point is that descriptive diagnoses are not helpful and offer no method for location or treatment. A proper diagnosis must have a structure listed to guide a treatment program. If an explanation is desired for any additional term, drop us a line and we will respond.

Chapter 3
How Pain is Diagnosed

As we discussed in the first chapter pain is an inflammatory change and has a source, which is an injured structure, and an endpoint, where you perceive the pain by an electrical impulse from that injured area. The brain tells you where the pain originates and how severe it is. Therefore no pain can be imagined or changed in any way due to emotion and/or psychological factors. Pain from any source is diagnosable primarily on a clinical basis, which is an examination by your doctor, which if done properly, will show a restricted movement which is the manifestation of the pain. When the movement of that body part is increased to normal, then that is the end point of diagnosis and treatment.

In order to do an adequate, indicated clinical examination of the musculoskeletal system, knowledge of the anatomy of the musculoskeletal system, including bone structure, muscle, nerves, tendons, ligaments, and joint capsules, and how all these parts work together, is absolutely necessary. This is what we call the normal physiology of weight bearing. This concept underlies every movement and every action. Pain is a failure of this physiology of weight bearing. There is no test available to indicate where pain arises. This includes all of the X-Ray procedures including MRI. The only test that can show us inflammation in a living body is the bone scan. The results however are subject to interpretation but do give you some objective findings on which to work. The physicians at Pain Centers. Nationwide (www.paintreatment.cc) are experts at the normal and abnormal physiology of weight bearing. The surgical anatomy, as practiced by very well-trained surgeons, is not the same as physiology as practiced by musculoskeletal physicians. My advice is to be treated by a musculoskeletal physician skilled in physiology, before considering treatment through surgery.

A specialized musculoskeletal history will concentrate on where the pain is and what motions produce it. We are not interested if pain is present all day. We are interested in specific questions, such as if the pain is produced by activities such as standing, walking, or arising. Specific activities reflect functioning of certain structures and not others. You may be surprised that lifting is not a specific activity we ask about because it is a culmination of the other activities.

The clinical exam is dictated by the history obtained from the patient. The patient is examined and any restriction of motion is recorded, with the normal physiology of motion and physiology of weight bearing in mind. The physiology of motion is the guiding principle of any examination. Any restriction of motion is the result of the painful structure. Since we know the pain patterns and where the restriction of motion occurs, we can then determine which structure is causing pain.

The neck, or cervical spine, has 6 main motions, and the back, or lumbar spine, has 4 main motions. The thoracic or dorsal spine in the rib area has 6 motions as well. The other joints have their normal ranges of motion which are assessed and these values can be found in any book. All aspects of the clinical exam are recorded as to degree of motion at which the pain is elicited. The side of pain elicitation and the degrees of motion are recorded and is the baseline data on which to judge any future improvement. We ask for a pain pattern and referral area, but we do not depend on what the patient says necessarily, instead how the patient examines.

We follow the clinical examination with a special weight bearing film which can reveal the history of all previous injuries and how to approach the painful area. The program we develop for each patient is based on the history and clinical examination, with the specific x-ray telling us how to approach that injured structure. This method individualizes the treatments for all patients. Spinal pain does not occur from front to back, but does occur from side to side. Think about that. If you look at the spine model, it is quite evident that the middle of the vertebra is solid bone, incapable of producing pain. The pain can only come from a moveable structure, therefore side to side because the moveable structures are located there. This was proven a long time ago in my clinical practice. Facets, nerves and discs are all lateralized. Normally, the spine can bear weight that is physical stress, because the stress is dissipated bilaterally on all of the structures of the spine. If one component is restricted, that is injured, then mobility is then decreased secondary to pain. In other words, motion is two sided. This fact is paramount to diagnosing the source of pain in the spine and other joints of the body, including shoulders, hips and knees.

The initial clinical examination is the baseline to judge all treatment and its success or failure. Improvement of motion is the goal, and this is an objective measure anyone can find. In contrast to this is the typical methods currently used, like the Visual Analog Scale, Short Form 36 (SF-36), and other subjective pain questionnaires. These are subjective and offer no method of verification. Science is based on objectivity, so it is difficult to reason why these methods remain in use. Subjective measures open the door for fraud, worker's compensation abuse, and legitimize narcotic addiction. There has been a recent article which criticized the use of these subjective tests, but this revolution of thought is still years away.

I would be extremely careful about accepting the notion of "neuropathic pain." There is no rationale for this concept. If a nerve is compromised as to its function, then there are appropriate tests to determine if the compromise is actually there. The motor branch and the sensory branch for each nerve in the body can be examined separately. There is no separation between axial pain and neuropathic pain. The pain is the same sensation. Motion decrease is the key to diagnosing pain. I am astonished at my colleagues who espouse the notion of the nerve system causing pain on its own for its own sake. This reasoning turns the science of anatomy and physiology on its head. When I ask these so called experts about the clinical findings, there is silence, and in the literature, you cannot find a decent history and clinical examination based on the normal physiology. In other words, the results of the research many times do not have a good history and clinical examination as a baseline for the research outcomes.

The basic approach we use to diagnose and treat pain is to encourage the patient to commit to a pain to be treated. I will in turn commit to treating that pain source. This is a bond between patient and physician which will produce the best results. This is an examination by committment.

Chapter 4
Neck Pain and Headache

When thinking about cervical pain before writing this chapter it becomes clear that there are so many interpretations of symptoms that an individual may have from various causes like acute trauma, small work-related injuries, or just working at home. All of these symptoms are in a continuum from mild, occasional stiffness to extreme pain to the point of immobility, but all symptoms are derived from the same structures. We need to look at these structures as more or less injured because there are no other structures there.

As a physician and consumer of health care, when I talk about an injury I am referring to an injured structure that can be treated. It is amazing to me that when I reviewed the medical literature for this book, the detail that I have included in this chapter is not in material available currently. For example, there are lists of information in other texts but there is no detail on how to approach a problem, how to examine it and definitely no instruction on how to treat it. There is no information on structures or why and where they are painful. There was an article published in 1990 that referenced the pain patterns of facet joint capsules, which is accurate, except we have included the lower facet of C_7-T_1 and the T_{1-2} as well. It was nice to see validation of the work we had honed over the 15 years prior to it. More importantly we have included an examination that takes these pain patterns into consideration.

I want you to read this chapter very closely because it is a protection for you to judge if you are being treated properly if you have a headache or neck pain. Remember there is no chronic pain requiring narcotics or mind-altering drugs. In essence you will learn more in this chapter to protect yourself than what most physicians, chiropractors, or physical therapists know.

The neck has seven vertebrae or bones, usually aligned with a slight lordosis, or front-to-back curve. The first two bones have a more specialized role in neck motion. The first bone, also called the atlas, on which the skull rests, has two important joints that allow nodding-like motion mainly with other motion patterns like rotation and side bend more restricted. The second bone, called the axis, has a large process that extends upward and creates an axis for the head and neck to rotate around. About one-half of the total rotation of a person's neck occurs at this level, with essentially no side bend or flexion-extension movements. The third through seventh cervical bones allow more generalized movement based on their anatomy. Refer to the drawing for more information. The neck bones are held together by two joints in the back, the facet joints, with their joint capsule ligament structure and the annulus, or disc, which is a specialized compound ligament that allows the variable motion that we all enjoy. There are 14 facet joints, 7 left-sided and 7 right-sided and 7 discs in the neck. The joints allow a person to look down and also to the left or right. The disc allows an individual to look upward and also to the left or right. There are muscles around the neck bones which pull the bones into the desired motion pattern. The muscles move the bones through a normal range of motion which is limited by the ligament structure. The ligaments prevent an excessive motion, though when there is an excessive force and this normal range of motion is exceeded, the result is an injury to the ligament structure primarily. The muscles may be injured as well though this is secondarily and less severe. This ligament injury is the source of most painful conditions.

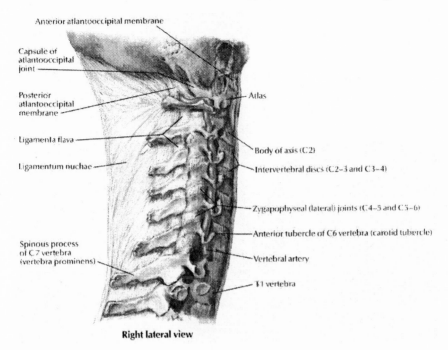

Anterior atlantooccipital membrane

Capsule of
atlantooccipital
joint

Posterior
atlantooccipital
membrane

Ligamenta flava

Ligamentum nuchae

Spinous process
of C7 vertebra
(vertebra prominens)

Atlas

Body of axis (C2)

Intervertebral discs (C2–3 and C3–4)

Zygapophyseal (lateral) joints (C4–5 and C5–6)

Anterior tubercle of C6 vertebra (carotid tubercle)

Vertebral artery

T1 vertebra

Right lateral view

View of the neck from the right side. Note the facet (zygapophyseal) joints in the back of the neck and the discs actually in the middle of the neck.

Nerves overall are not an important part of the "cervical syndrome" or pain in the neck. Remember as we discussed before a nerve compromise causes a tingle and/or sensory loss in a particular area. Nerve injuries in the neck will have upper limb symptoms in the specific area for that nerve root.

The cervical spine moves in 6 prime motions: flexion-extension, left and right lateral rotation, left and right lateral bending. Flexion is touching the chin to the chest and extension is raising the chin into the air. Rotation refers to putting the chin on the respective shoulder. Lateral bending refers to putting the ear on the shoulder.

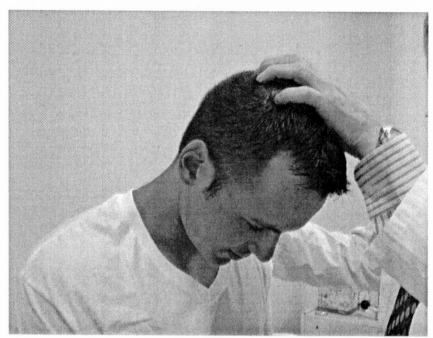

Cervical flexion, touching the chin to the chest.

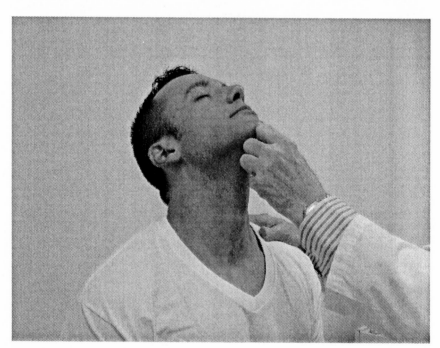

Cervical extension, raising the chin.

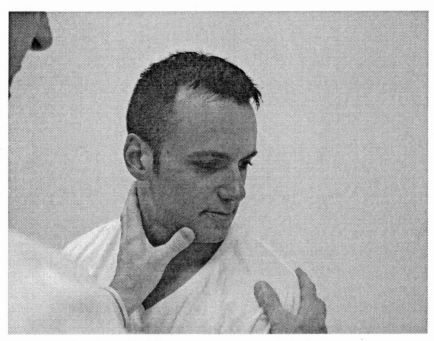

Left lateral rotation, putting the chin on the left shoulder.

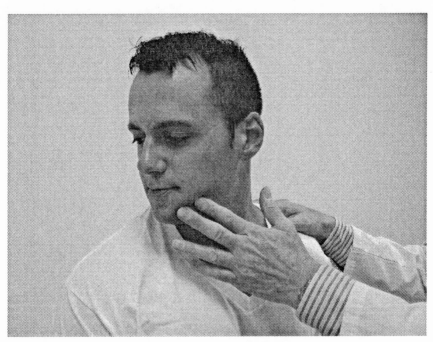

Right lateral rotation, putting the chin on the right shoulder.

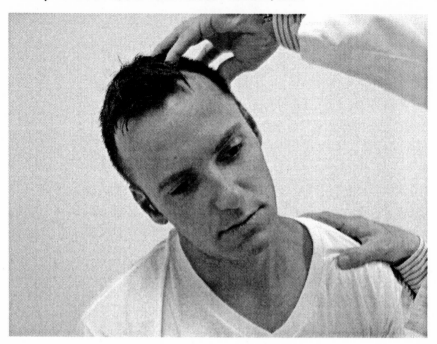

Right lateral bend, putting the right ear on the shoulder

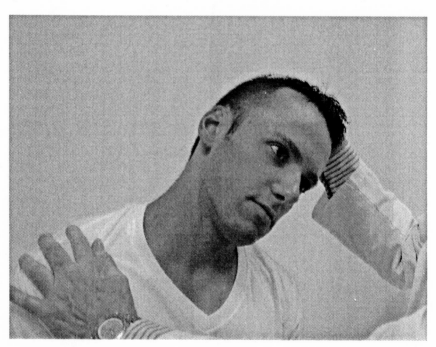

Left lateral bend, putting the left ear on the shoulder.

The cervical spine has the most movement in the upper levels, with the most movement in the first three segments as it attaches to the skull. This allows most of the head movements. The remainder of the cervical spine is designed to allow maximal motion of the head, lateral rotation to 90 degrees and neck extension to 40 degrees or so. Any injury of the ligament structure will cause a decreased movement in one or more of these six prime motions. The bone and ligament structure allow the normal movements and any injury to the ligament structure causes a decrease in the normal movement with a typical pain pattern.

If these six motions are equal side-to-side without pain, there is no cervical source present. The history must be specific enough to lead the examiner to the source of that pain. The examination verifies the history and will be able to determine the decreased movement in the prime motions, which reflects on the injured structures unable to move. This is how a diagnosis is to be made. This is also how a recheck examination or examination for fakery should be performed. If the motion is normal there is no source of pain in the neck.

The cervical structures causing pain have already been described to you above, but they are the facet joint capsules, annulus, and muscle-bone connector. If there is a pain in the shoulder or trapezius muscle, the pain is from the C_{4-5} level. If there is no pain in the trapezius or upper back with moving the neck the painful source is higher in the neck, at C_{3-4}, C_{2-3}, C_{1-2}, or C_0-C_1. This will include many undiagnosed sources of headache and face pain. Any pain of the neck also involving the shoulder muscles must involve structures at or below C_{4-5}. As just mentioned the C_{4-5} level will refer to the upper trapezius muscle as well as the eyeball. The C_{5-6} level will refer to the shoulder blade, slightly lower and more to the shoulder joint than the C_{4-5} level. The C_{6-7} level will refer along side the shoulder blade in the middle of the back and C_7-T_1 refers lower than C_{6-7}. Refer to the illustration. All the referral patterns listed above are from the facet joints. The illustration below was taken from a 1990 publication which concurs with what we worked out years before.

37

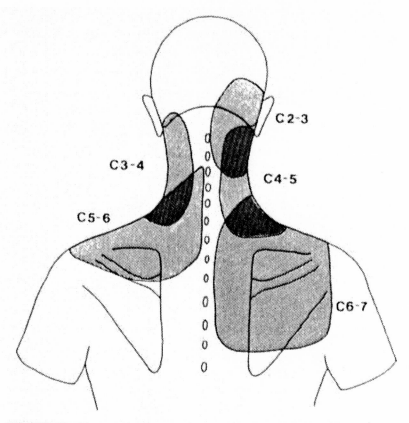

FIGURE 37–23. Pain referral from C2 to C3 through C6 to C7 facet joints. (From Dwyer A, Aprill C, Bogduk N: Cervical zygapophyseal joint pain patterns. I. A study in normal volunteers. Spine 1990; 15:456.)

The annulus is another structure in the middle of the neck which refer to the front of the face, neck, and upper chest depending on which levels are involved. The annulus will cause pain in a similar pattern as the facet joints, though the examination will be different because raising the chin will provoke the pain rather than lowering it. Nerves have a specific pain pattern. The fifth cervical nerve, C_5, has a neck pain with referral over the side of the shoulder, but the shoulder is not painful on moving the joint. The sixth cervical nerve, C_6, goes to the forearm and/or thumbs and causes a tingling sensation. The seventh nerve, C_7, goes to the back of the arm and causes a tingling in the index and long fingers. The eighth cervical nerve, C_8, goes to the back of the arm and causes a tingle to the little and ring fingers.

There is another syndrome concerning the neck pain with referral to the upper limb. The "strap" muscles, or scalene muscles, cause pain under the shoulder blade and into the arm but does not have a specific nerve component. These muscles are in the front of the neck and act as guide wires as they pull the head from side to side. There will be tenderness along the first rib where these muscles attach. The evaluation of this syndrome must begin above T_6.

We need to discuss the mechanisms of injuries for the structures that we describe. Injuries can be sports injuries, falling down steps, automobile crashes, digging stumps out at home, cleaning the house, and so on. There is no specific injury that can occur at work that is different than an injury from any other cause or place. Why? Because there are only so many structures that can be injured in the human body. We will have more on work-related injuries in another chapter. Referring back to the automobile accident, it is said that if the car does not incur too much damage, then how can those inside it be injured? The defense against the insurance company is that the injury the occupant receives does not equate to the injury of the automobile, because the severity of the person's injury depends on several factors. One is the previous state of health. The second is the way the occupant was sitting. Was the person sitting on the left buttock or right buttock, or looking straight ahead or looking up or down, or to the right or left? The maximum forces on the cervical spine depend on how the structures were aligned on impact which is only a fraction of a second. Injuries can only be examined by a history and examination, not by how much damage was done to the car. The worst type of injury is the rear-ender because of the rapid acceleration and deceleration of the head and the chance the head can hit the wheel or windshield.

The next type of injury would be the lifting injury, when trying to lift something heavy and using the neck to help lift. This can affect the neck and other parts of the spine and hips. If you lift without bending your arms at the elbow, the force of the object is transmitted to the cervical spine. See the illustrations for this type of mechanism.

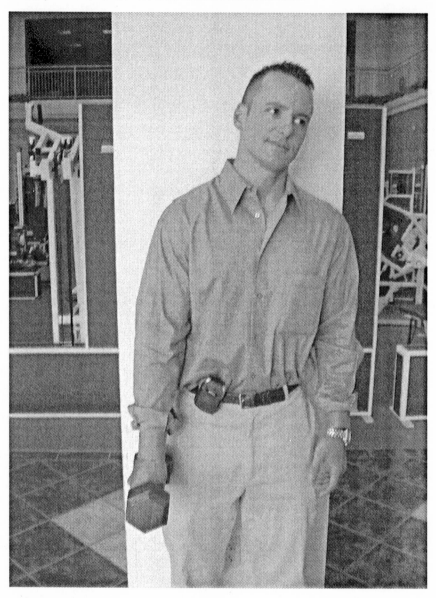

Lifting an object with a straight elbow transmits force to the neck, which may injure structures there.

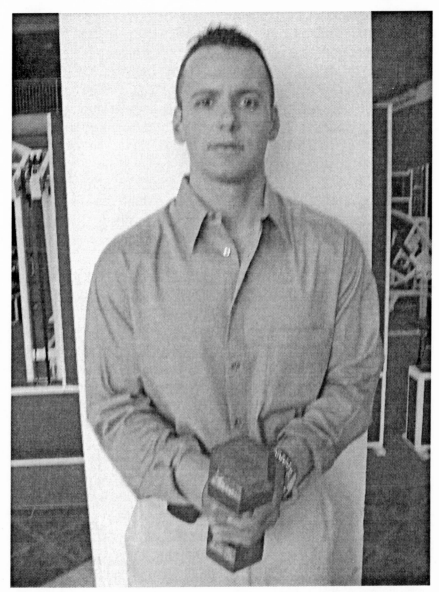

Lifting an object with the elbows bent lessens the chance for neck injury.

This tends to lead to muscular injuries along the side of the neck, specifically the "strap" muscles where they attach to the first rib. I know this because the prime motions of the neck, flexion, extension, etc. are usually intact after injuries such as this. I generally have not

41

seen cervical annular injuries from lifting in my 35 years of practice. The pain will resolve in only a few days if it is the muscle itself that is painful, though it can linger if the tendon structure is the culprit. The individual should restrict lifting until the pain resolves.

The backpack injury is also a cervical injury, with a thoracic component. Looking up for any prolonged period of time will stretch the anterior ligament structure or annulus and cause symptoms. All of these pain syndromes involve the same structures except they decrease in severity. They can be diagnosed by history and clinical examination.

Starting with the history of the pain pattern and the activity which produces that pain and special film to instruct us on how to approach the problem, an individual program will be outlined for fast, permanent improvement. Pain needs to be lateralized with a source. The examiner should be skilled enough to gain this information through a history and clinical examination, as we are at Pain Centers. Nationwide (www.paintreatment.cc).

Painful neck flexion, or touching the chin to the chest, will usually be from facet joint capsules. You can treat this at home yourself by using ear-to-shoulder motions, which seems to reset the bone structure and equalizes the motion of the joint capsules on each side, thus relieving the pain. You may try to adjust the pillows while lying down to get the stretch off the painful joint. Anti-inflammatories, such as aspirin and the like, are always recommended. The important things to look for are continued stiffness and the inability to raise your chin. We do not recommend hot-packs or ice-packs at home because they are ineffective. If the stiffness is too great, that it begins to interfere with home life or working, we recommend formal treatment including ultrasound, traction, extension exercises, and oral medications. No treatment however, will be effective if a proper and complete diagnosis is not established at the onset.

We use 6 types of cervical traction depending on the diagnosis of the offending structure. Headache at the base of the skull is treated by cervical traction in the supine position. Joint pain is treated by what I call joint stretch, again depending on which joint is involved and which side is the primary structure is to be mobilized. The lower structures in the neck are treated by what I call side push which will only mobilize these lower structures. Annular pain is treated this way along with facetal structures. Very young patients may not need traction because their ligaments are supple enough that they can be mobilized. Older patients, especially those patients who have had a very physically demanding history with many injuries, or those whose ligaments are really stiff can benefit from these techniques. If the pain and stiffness is too great and the range of motion is severely restricted, and the lifestyle of the patient is affected, then the offending structure can be injected with a small amount of steroid for Pannozzo's ten minute test regime. If relief is obtained in 10 minutes and the range of motion is returned, then the next day that pain will not be present.

We have developed the technique of injecting not only the facets, but also the annulus if found to be painful. If a nerve is involved, as diagnosed by EMG, then the facet and annulus on that side can be injected, and the tissues mobilized to relieve that nerve. The idea of injecting the facets was taught to me by Dr. Maigne in a class that he gave many years ago. Because of my patient load, I was able to expand the technique to include the facets and annulus and to produce the protocol for evaluation and treatment. There are many details to this scenario that cannot be included here. When evaluating a neck pain and headache, the upper dorsal spine to T_6 must be included because a curvature there will affect the side to side curvature of the neck. If not straight, then adequate weight bearing cannot be accomplished, and a pain will appear. Some of the chronic and untreatable cervical pain can be based on this fact.

As far as treatments are concerned, without a proper diagnosis, none will predictably be effective for you. Physical therapy using hot or cold packs cannot be effective in the short or long run. Chiropractic manipulation likewise cannot isolate an individual structure to be treated and is too rough in my opinion. I have studied osteopathic and chiropractic techniques but do not use them. Perhaps a stretching regime is more useful, if the diagnosis can be localized. Alternative treatment of diet and yoga and Pilates and the myriad fads going on today cannot do you any good because those promulgating these techniques are not skilled in diagnosis, therefore, how do they know what they are doing. I am not saying for you not do those regimes, but if you want your pain to be gone, then think about it. For headache then, the dietary restrictions bandied about are not based on fact.

I recently had the privilege of a 34 year old woman who suffered from cervical pain and headache for 8 months with headache at the back of the head on the right. She was unable to be seen in my office because her insurance company would not allow this under her policy. She switched insurance coverage so that she could see me. The treatments that she undertook before seeing me consisted of chiropractic manipulation, physical therapy and Flexeril. The MRI showed many abnormalities but none stood out except for compression of the disc at C_{4-5} and C_{6-7}. No lateralization was given. On the clinical examination, there was a restricted motion of the cervical spine especially on flexion of a loss of 10 degrees and extension, with a loss of 10 degrees. The trapezius muscle pain produced on the left, only. The C_{4-5} facet and annulus on the left was the main painful structure verified by palpation, after my film was taken and reviewed, showing the left side was the main side to treat. The headache was coming from the C_{1-2} area on the right. Treatment options were explained to the patient. She chose the injection method. The injections were placed at the facet and annulus of the left C_{4-5} level. After 10 minutes, she was reexamined. Now the movement of the neck in flexion and extension was completely normal without pain. The headache was treated by a special mobilization technique that I developed. Her headache was gone! This is what the patient stated for the record. This was the Pannozzo 10 minute test, which predicts a cure by the next day, the pain not to return. I wanted to site this medical case as the routine evaluation and treatment for the neck pain and headache. This rapid reduction of the main documented symptoms and signs of the painful condition is what you want for treatment of your cervical pain and headache. This approach can be found, but not easily. This type of approach is used in the treatment of all painful conditions any place in the body.

Another patient to illustrate the cervical phenomenon is as follows: A 63 year old lady presented to me the problem of weakness of the left shoulder of 6 months duration. She was unable to lift the arm to the side away from the body. She could sleep on it, however. She was given meds for pain and sent to the physical therapist. He referred her back to the doctor for a shot. When I examined her, there was no restriction of motion, but weakness of the supraspinatus muscle was quite evident. The neck was examined, showing a lack of extension but no pain was elicited into the shoulder. The possibilities at this time were avulsion of the tendon or a nerve root motor branch malfunction. An EMG was done in my office, and x-ray of the neck was done and shoulder film was read. The EMG showed a C_6 radiculopathy, motor branch. The film was read to show us how to proceed with our treatment. The annulus and facet on that side was treated, and a dorsal concavity was treated, resulting in a large percentage of discomfort being reduced. No medications were need except aspirin. This case scenario illustrates a full service musculoskeletal pain clinic and the rapid response to pain that can be achieved. This is physician treatment at its best. We do not waste time with physical therapy, chiropractic, or any other non-direct ways to treat patients.

As far as the notion of the patient faking symptoms from an auto accident or other trauma, the emotional, and psychiatric, or psychological evaluation should not be a consideration. There is a consideration for sick leave if the job cannot be done because of physical stress, and if the ROM exam is normal or not. When the normal range of motion of the neck is achieved without pain, then the case is concluded. Steady progress to that end is made in the course of the treatment.

As far as treatments are concerned, if a neck pain is mild and early, then based on the special x-ray, treatments with ultra sound to a specified area is accomplished along with oral medication of an anti inflammatory nature, and a home exercise of stretching is given. If the pain is more severe and headache is present, then we may want to add cervical traction-one of the 6-8 types we offer. If the pain and headache causes so much pain that motion is lost, and the life style and work is affected, then the facetal and annular injections are offered. At no time are narcotic drugs given.

Headache and Migraine Headache

Headache is an entirely different subject and this should be read several times because it will be very important. One of the major syndromes of neck pain is headache. A headache is a referred pain from a pulled ligament structure, which is a bone-to-bone connector.

Much of the research I performed on headache was done on myself and thousands of patients. I found that if a throbbing headache is present, it may be relieved temporarily by putting the head back, thereby relaxing the tension on the joint capsules. Another patient had eyeball pain and neck pain upon flexion. By doing a careful examination I found that the C_{4-5} facet on the painful side was tender. Knowing that there was only one joint that was painful, I proposed to the patient about injecting that particular joint. Ten minutes after the injection the eyeball pain subsided and the cervical examination improved. This immediate success started me on the long quest of isolating all the structures in the neck and categorizing their pain patterns and then relating all headaches to this.

There are different types of headaches described in the literature today: 1. Cluster headache, a one-sided usually short duration pain that is typically around the eye and may occur several times per day. 2. Migraine headache, a throbbing pain that tends to last for several hours and progresses from one-sided to diffuse. The person may experience difficulty with light and may have an "aura" or some symptoms that tend to precede the onset of the migraine. 3. Tension-type headache, a diffuse, band-like moderate intensity pain, not described as pulsating and does not cause nausea, and usually no difficulties with normal light or sounds.

The cause of these different types of headaches is still controversial in the neurology literature. For many years it was felt that migraine headache was related to an abnormal blood-flow pattern in the brain, however that did not explain all the symptoms that migraine sufferers feel. Later other thoughts emerged, ranging from various brain changes to different chemical interactions to a "migraine center"—none have been proven thus far. The causes behind cluster headache are even less understood, with theories of brain hormone imbalances and immune system disorders as potential reasons. Tension-type headaches are now felt to not be caused by tension at all—instead abnormal neuronal sensitivity in combination with several chemical and hormonal imbalances. It is interesting that the more these pains are investigated, the less sure anyone is about the cause and instead more theories and imbalances and disorders get described. As a consumer of health care I would like to impress upon you the concept of the mechanism, or how something causes pain. For example it is recommended to avoid alcohol around the time of a cluster headache because it may elicit a pain, though how it would do this is unclear. What I notice is that when drinking alcohol the person tends to raise the chin to get the beer at the bottom of the bottle, or the last few ounces of wine in the glass. This neck motion causes a stress on some of the ligament structures in the neck, which will not be immediately perceived due to the effects of the alcohol. The next day headache will be perceived and be blamed on the alcohol, but is due to the ligament structures. To prove this scenario to myself I have treated people with day-after headaches from drinking and have always found a painful structure in the neck. We treat these areas with physical medicine technique and the headache disappears.

Since the types of headache are not defined and theories constantly change, you should be alerted as I am that there is no science in the treatment of headache based on those ideas. I view headache as having two possible sources: 1) In the brain, like a tumor or aneurysm 2.) External to the brain, as in the cervical spine. Today it is very easy to find if there is a brain lesion causing headache, which is by CT scan. It is well worth the money to show a brain lesion is not present. If there is no tumor in the brain, then the headache must be coming from the neck primarily.

The symptoms of headache are 1. Throbbing sensation, which I have traced to the facet capsule. 2. Dull headache, which I have traced to the annulus. 3. There can be a combination of dull and throbbing, depending on which structures are most painful. The cervical spine has the most movement in the upper levels, with the most movement in the first three segments as it attaches to the skull. This allows most of the head movements. This is also the source of headache, a dull "migranous" type of head ache. Which facet or annulus is causing the pain is dependent upon the history and pain pattern and clinical exam which brings out the location of the painful structure. The special film tells us how to approach that structure. This is the approach I would want for my headache. We have treated people taking the best medication for years who were not helped. We were able to help them because we were able to offer an individual diagnosis and treatment based on the findings. We do not use the usual drugs and instead use physical means for treatment.

As mentioned earlier in the chapter, only certain neck levels refer pain to the head. We can postulate that the C_{4-5} level is the lowest level to refer pain to the head, and this refers toward the face and eyeball. The levels below this, like the C_{5-6} and C_{6-7} and lower, do not cause headache just refer pain toward the torso. The C_{3-4} level will refer up the side of the face and the up the back of the head, as will the C_{2-3}, C_{1-2}, and C_0-C_1. The C_0-C_1 and C_{1-2} levels are the cause of migraine I believe, because it fits the symptom pattern—one sided headache without referral lower in the neck. If you follow these rules you will be very happy with the reduction of your headache.

In the matter of migraine headache in particular we have determined that an accurate clinical examination of the top of the neck and at the base of the skull will reveal the source of this type of headache. Recall that it is based on the C_{1-2} and C_0-C_1 joints. One side is relatively fixed and one side is hypermobile, leading to ligament overstretch and pain. The pain can be either side, however. Treatment by mobilizing the tight side, which may be the opposite side of the pain, offers the best result. Any X-Ray taken for this purpose will show this fact, correlating to the headache (see example below). You can evaluate this yourself by putting your thumbs at the base of the skull and the top of the neck and feel for an area of and tightness on one side and an area of spacing and looseness on the other side. The area of tightness must be stretched accordingly to equal the other side. In this manner the headache will disappear over time without any drugs necessary. During the meantime we suggest you take several aspirin thirty minutes before you stretch your neck.

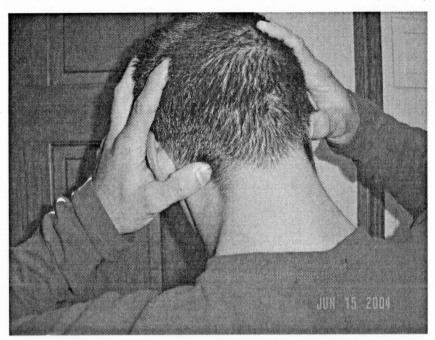

Place thumbs at base of skull to compare tightness and tenderness with the opposite site. This is the joint between the skull and the first neck bone.

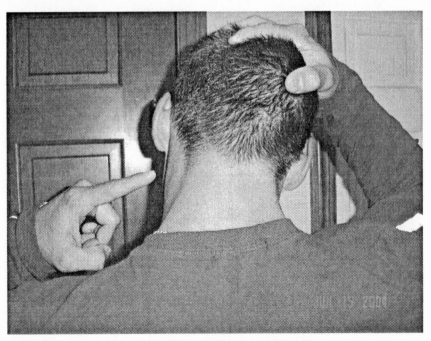

Stretch the tight side by pulling head to the opposite side.

49

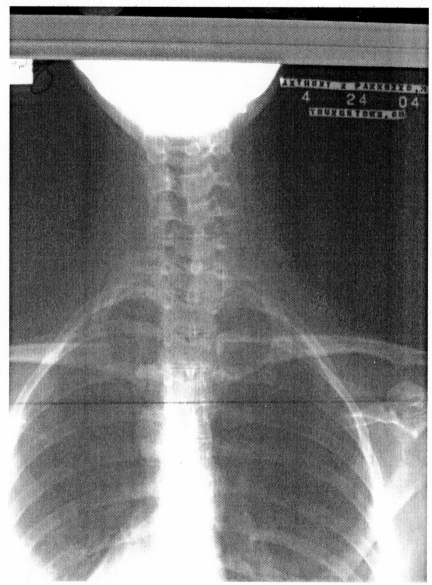

Film of a patient with chronic migraine headache. Notice how the neck curves to the left side due to tightness on that side. You can see just below the skull there is less spacing on the left side, which needs to be mobilized for relief.

The treatment for headache is quite easy if you have treated thousands of people like I have. I recall seeing a girl who had a headache for two days. My daughter asked me to look at her and went through the evaluation just described. By examination I found a painful level on the opposite side of the headache. I next went to the joint on the opposite side and mobilized it and the headache had disappeared after 10 minutes.

Many cases of Multiple Sclerosis are made by a diagnosis of face pain, which is related to the upper cervical spine. The reasons why these sources are missed are that there needs to be a suspicion of these injuries, and often the neck is just not examined. We know this to be true because patients tell us the previous examinations were not as comprehensive as ours. The best examination for the upper portions of the cervical spine is range of motion with palpation of the upper portions. What we are looking for is excessive motion on one side, which causes a headache. The excessive motion on one side is due to the swivel effect because of injury about the joint on the opposite side causing abnormally limited movement on the injured side. Any headache can give the photophobic effect and force a individual to lie down or have nausea and vomiting.

Knowing what I just described above, I can tell you the theory of headache as propounded by headache clinics and others who describe migraine as vascular in nature as patently false and unproven.

Here is a typical case of a 17 year-old male injured in a rear collision. At impact his head went backwards, causing neck pain and severe headache. He was treated for 6 months for headache before we saw him in our offices. During that time he was tested by X-Ray, EEG, and given treatments consisting of physical therapy, electrical stimulation, and weight lifting twice weekly for six weeks. The neck pain was especially prominent on the left side, radiating to the left temple and top of the shoulder. After examination we determined that the pain was most prominent from the C_{5-6} level on the right side, which was affecting higher levels in the neck. These higher levels in the neck were the source of the headache, but this was all related to the lower C_{5-6} level. These areas were treated by injecting the joint with total relief of that headache. We know this is true because he was seen for a back pain three months later, and he stated he no longer had neck pain or headache. This is a typical example of how we approach headache, with examination and specific treatment plan. Excellent results are rapidly obtained if the proper structure is treated.

Chapter 5
Shoulder Pain

I hope you read this chapter several times because there is a great deal of information and misinformation available for us all to read. In general there is a mystery about shoulders and shoulder injuries and a great deal of controversy on how to treat them. From 1996 to 1999 I have successfully treated 980 shoulders. Therefore I am supremely qualified to give my opinions on how to go about this.

The shoulder is comprised of three joints:

1. The ball-and-socket-like glenohumeral joint, what is generally described as the shoulder.
2. The acromioclavicular joint, where the acromion, which is part of the scapula or shoulder blade, and the clavicle, or collar bone, meet.
3. The scapulothoracic joint, which is not what most would consider a true joint. The scapula, or shoulder blade, floats on the structures of the back and has an important role in total shoulder mobility.

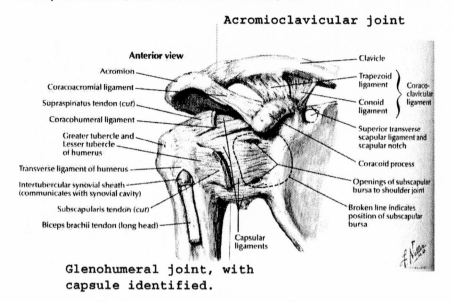

Acromioclavicular joint

Anterior view

Acromion

Coracoacromial ligament

Supraspinatus tendon (cut)

Coracohumeral ligament

Greater tubercle and Lesser tubercle of humerus

Transverse ligament of humerus

Intertubercular synovial sheath (communicates with synovial cavity)

Subscapularis tendon (*cut*)

Biceps brachii tendon (long head)

Clavicle

Trapezoid ligament } Coraco-clavicular ligament

Conoid ligament

Superior transverse scapular ligament and scapular notch

Coracoid process

Openings of subscapular bursa to shoulder joint

Broken line indicates position of subscapular bursa

Capsular ligaments

Glenohumeral joint, with capsule identified.

The glenohumeral joint, like all joints, has a capsule covering which accommodates motion of the joint through a normal amount of flexibility. The capsule of the shoulder joint goes from the arm bone, or humerus, to the opposite side of the joint the glenoid portion of the scapula. This is where most of the motion occurs in the joint. This capsule has a nerve supply and is a major pain producing structure if its usual flexibility is compromised. The acromioclavicular joint has a capsule similar to this also. The capsular ligament allows a normal amount of motion but inhibits excessive motion. This is why we are not "double-jointed". The shoulder joint, capsule, and muscles have nerve supply from the C_5 and C_6 nerves from the neck.

The muscles of the shoulder attach via tendons to create the marvelous motions we all know. The main muscle group is the "rotator cuff", which is made of four separate muscles. The main component of the rotator cuff is the supraspinatus muscle, which is the prime mover for the arm bone to be raised from the side, bringing the elbow upward. The supraspinatus is the muscle that is most often referred to as being torn on an MRI. Another important muscle group is the teres muscle group. These muscles are located in the back of the shoulder blade. The teres minor muscle specifically extends to the back of the arm bone and is a frequent source of pain.

There is a surgical approach and a non-surgical approach to shoulder injuries. There are various terms applied to shoulder injuries. The most commonly used is rotator cuff syndrome or cuff tear. This term could imply to you that there was a real tear, as in a piece of paper, of the structure. In actuality that is not true. Breakages of muscle are self-limited and they heal and they do not have to be operated unless the tendon is avulsed or pulled off of the bone or there is a total (100%) tear and the arm is not able to be raised to the side. In my experience the tear of the rotator cuff is not causing the pain. Instead, the pain is localized to the capsule or to the supraspinatus tendon insertion. The tear, if there is one, must cause blood loss, because muscle is a very vascular and active tissue. This blood loss can only be diagnosed by MRI. However, the MRI cannot tell you where the pain arises. It must be interpreted by clinical examination, and you are subject to the skills of the examiner. So be careful. So to recap then, if a rotator cuff tear is diagnosed, but is causing pain in the capsule or at the supraspinatus insertion, or shows no blood leakage on the MRI, then it is probably not a symptomatic rotator cuff tear and can be treated by non-surgical methods. In order for this to be treated though, the source of pain must be diagnosed. We separate the shoulder into functional units. For instance, we separate the ligament structure that holds the bones together from the muscular structure with its tendons that actually move the bones. We have devised a simple exam which takes into consideration the anatomy and physiology and design of the shoulder joint.

Hold the elbow away from the body as much as 90 degrees if possible. If this is painful, it indicates restriction of the joint capsule in the axilla, or under part of the shoulder. If you rotate the wrist upward toward the ceiling, it examines the front of the shoulder capsule. Lowering the wrist toward the floor examines the back of the shoulder capsule. If those motions are painful, the appropriate joint capsule, or ligament structure, needs to be treated and the pain problem is not the rotator cuff. Holding the arm outward at 90° and resisting applied pressure to the elbow tests the rotator cuff tendon, primarily the supraspinatus muscle tendon. If there is strength of this tendon without pain, you do not have a rotator cuff problem. This exam will tell you approximately where your problems are so that you can get treated properly. If you cannot sleep on a shoulder, it is because the joint capsule cannot stretch to accommodate this sleep position. Proper treatment for these injuries is to stretch the capsule and strengthen the tendon. Anti-inflammatory medications are helpful for this. If you cannot sleep on this shoulder because of pain, or cannot work, or you just want the pain removed, we can by this good exam locate the pain and inject that area with a steroid and pain killer. The usual 10 minute test takes place.

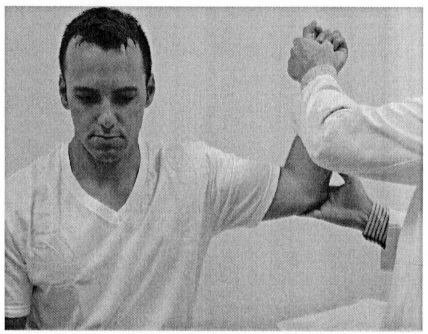

Passive external rotation of the glenohumeral joint.

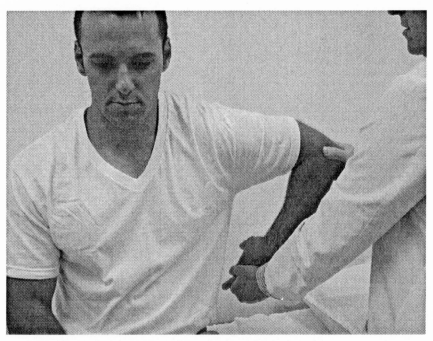

Passive internal rotation of the glenohumeral joint.

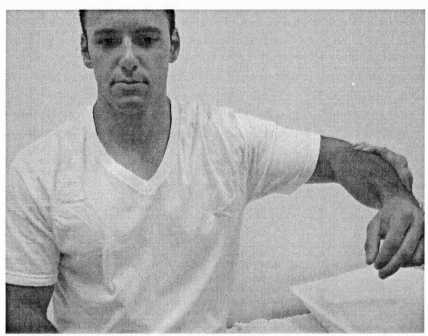

Resisted abduction, testing primarily the supraspinatus muscle, the major muscle of the "rotator cuff".

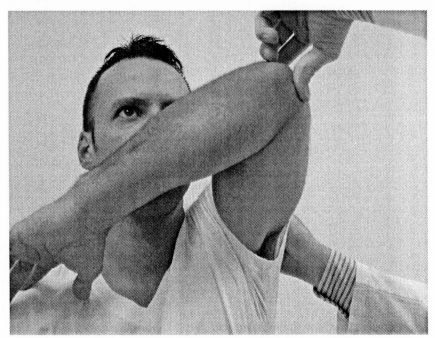

Testing for the acromioclavicular joint, where the collar bone meets the shoulder.

The next important part of the shoulder is the acromioclavicular joint, or AC joint. For this exam, place your hand on the opposite shoulder and raise your elbow. If this is painful, then the acromioclavicular joint is the injured part of the shoulder and must be treated. This little ligament is usually treated by injection procedure, though it can be treated by a stretching maneuver and ultrasound.

If you cannot sleep on your shoulder, the pain is capsular, or ligamentous, in origin. This would be diagnosed as limited range of motion due to pain as described before. This does not require physical therapy and does not require surgery or chiropractic treatment. If the stretching program does not relive the pain, the area of the capsule responsible for the pain should be isolated by physical exam and injected.

If you do not make a rapid improvement, then the diagnosis, as we might expect, is not accurate. There is no shoulder that should be operated if the techniques above are followed.

There is reference in the literature to the unstable shoulder joint, or the hypermobile shoulder joint. Our approach to this is to identify a tight area of the shoulder, which does not have the normal mobility. Our treatments are aimed at improving this immobility and restoring normal function overall. We do not treat the hyper mobile part of the joint capsule as this is already stretched. Some practitioners will want to tighten this part of the joint capsule; this is not an approach I use. We do mobilize the restricted part of the joint capsule, thereby allowing the loosened part to reposition itself, and tighten by itself, to normal. The anterior and posterior shoulder capsule can be mobilized by specific exercise. The exercise to stretch the posterior capsule is to bring the arm across the chest, holding the elbow with the opposite hand. The anterior capsule is mobilized by rotating the arm outward with the palm pointing upward. See the pictures below.

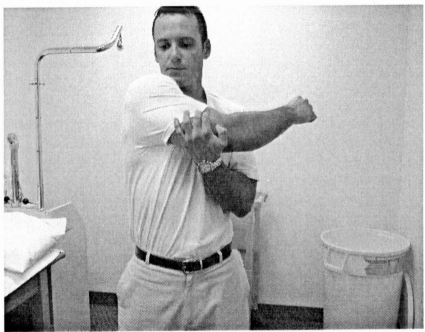

The posterior shoulder capsule is stretched by bringing the arm across the chest and holding the back of the elbow with the opposite hand.

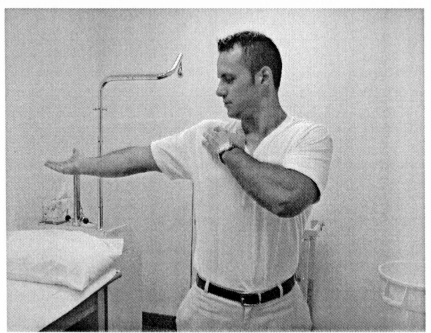

The anterior capsule is mobilized by turning the palm upward and rotating the arm outward. The stretch should be felt where the model is pointing.

There is reference to labrum injuries, for example SLAP lesions, and others. I believe that these are merely a part of the capsule and cannot be distinguished. They are treated in similar fashion to anterior capsular injuries.

Impingement syndrome is manifested as pain in the front of the shoulder when bringing the arm forward and across the body. This is due to tightness of the posterior capsule. If the back of the shoulder does not stretch out properly in the back, it kinks in the front thereby producing pain. Treatment for this is mobilization of the posterior capsule.

The teres muscle can also be painful but is differentiated by having a normal capsule examination. This is usually treated with ultrasound. What I use in my clinic after ultrasound is a technique I call minimobilization. This simple technique is effective in mobilizing a ligament, but the location must be secure before it will be effective.

The Teres major and minor muscle insertion into the humerous bone can cause a tingling sensation to the hand to the little finger side. This can be a very painful shoulder and could be misdiagnosed as a cervical nerve problem. The difference in diagnosis is that the shoulder will ache, and the range of motion of the shoulder joint will be normal, and the neck will examine normal too. If necessary, an EMG can be done. However, palpation of one shoulder and then the other for comparison and testing the strength of the muscle, will elicit the localization of the enthesitis causing syndrome. The ten minute test by injection will give fast almost complete relief and thus the diagnosis is secure. This injury can take place in the gym, or other pulling exercises or chores.

The usual treatments such as climbing the wall with your hand, ice and hotpacks, and an exercise program for strength by a physical therapist in an orthopedic surgeon's office will be a failure in most cases. Failed treatments generally lead to an MRI, but patients should be wary because MRIs are mostly over-read and this read can lead directly to the operating room. Be careful of surgery to the shoulder. The result of surgical intervention is a scar across the top of the glenohumeral joint that will be painful and with decreased function for a long time.

We use local steroid injection into the damaged ligament structure only. There is no reason to inject the inside of the shoulder joint. The pain and calcium formation as a repair of a damaged shoulder is strictly outside the shoulder and not in the synovium or lining of the joint. The orthopedists who I know continue to inject long acting steroids into the joint. This should be condemned for two reasons. One, the synovium is almost always normal. Two, long acting anything is not to be used because of the lack of sophistication and lack of control of the substance once injected. The last word is that the shoulder is easily treated without looking inside. Most pain is from the ligament structure and not the shoulder itself. Arthroscopic surgery has no advantage at all. Rotator cuff surgery makes no sense. Look at it this way—if there is a tear anywhere, of any significance, it is usually not painful at the tear, but at the insertion of the muscle at the humerus. This is the area to treat, and is readily accessible by a one half inch needle.

In my experience, MRIs are over read. Sometimes I feel they are read for the surgeon.

Chapter 6
Dorsal and Chest Pain

Pain below the neck and above the lumbar spine is what is called the thoracic or dorsal spine. See the illustration below which shows this part of the spine.

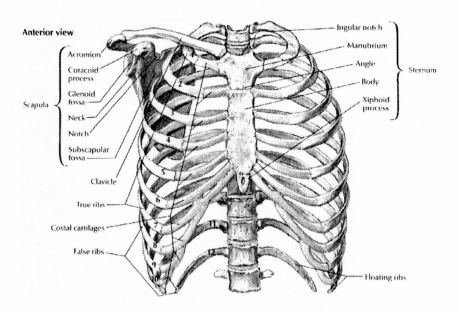

Anterior view

Acromion

Coracoid process

Glenoid fossa

Scapula

Neck

Notch

Subscapular fossa

Clavicle

True ribs

Costal cartilages

False ribs

Jugular notch

Manubrium

Angle

Body

Sternum

Xiphoid process

Floating ribs

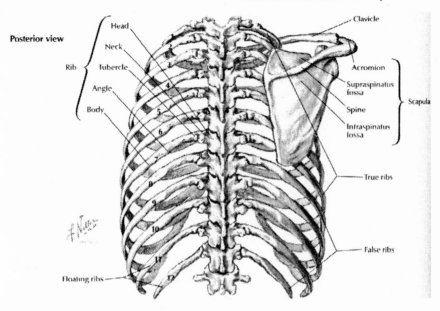

Posterior view

Head
Neck
Rib
Tubercle
Angle
Body
Floating ribs

Clavicle
Acromion
Supraspinatus fossa
Spine
Infraspinatus fossa
Scapula
True ribs
False ribs

This area of the spine has relevant structures which are the similar to the cervical or lumbar spine, as well as the unique rib cage structure. The ribs attach to the vertebral body itself and wrap around toward the front along a downward and lateral path. Muscles that make up the torso/chest wall attach to the ribs along their entire course. The ribs attach to cartilage toward the front of the chest. This cartilage continues and attaches to the sternum, or breastbone. The bone-cartilage junction is an important cause of pain, known commonly as *costo-chondritis*. Not to be overlooked, however, is the muscular insertion on the ribs, which is extremely common yet commonly missed.

The thoracic spine is stabilized by the rib cage. The facet joint orientation and the rib attachments limit the ability for the thoracic spine to flex and extend, though rotation is one of the primary motions of this area.

The vertebral body is solid bone and not a pain generator usually. It is connected to other vertebrae by joints and the joint capsules, which can be painful. The disc, or annulus, connects the front part of the vertebral bodies together, and in this part of the spine is usually not a pain generator. The disc in this area can be read as abnormal on an MRI scan, but this does not usually reflect the source of pain. In this part of the back, the joint capsule is the primary source of pain between the shoulder blades. Pain from this source can be severe or just a nag. This is also the site of most fibromyalgia pain.

The dorsal spine is also involved in scoliosis usually, and will produce the so-called "second curve". This curve in the dorsal spine can be primary, which is when one vertebral bone slides into the bone below which begins the abnormality. The spine will then be curved to the subluxed side, then curve toward the other side to correct itself above. If this does not take place, a person with scoliosis would walk crooked. Scoliosis can be this simple or part or a larger problem, with three or more curves, though this is handled in similar fashion. The subluxed side must be mobilized to straight. Treatment should be begun as fast as possible, otherwise permanent bone changes may result. Surgery should be seen as unnecessary if this approach is followed. The surgical approach for this entity is unnecessary. Our approach to this problem is to find the sources of the curve and then to mobilize the bone structure to normal position. The bone structure will remain in the normal position, thus eliminating the curvature. We have treated many of these cases, before surgery and after. Many rods have been removed and the patient rehabilitated to a normal pain free range of motion. There cannot be a genetic basis for scoliosis. We will have a chapter on this later.

What happens usually in instances of mid-back pain is a joint capsule on one side being over-stretched which causes a pain at that level. This is diagnosed by palpating the spine and finding the most tender area. Palpation can be performed in a seated or standing position. The tender area is located and after counting downward from the base of the neck a specific diagnosis can made. This then can be compared to the standing X-ray to evaluate the dorsal spine, and if any lower abnormality is causing the pain at the diagnosed level secondarily. What you need to know about a dorsal pain is that it needs to be treated as a two-sided problem. Though the pain may be only on one side, both sides must be treated for mobilization.

Pain patterns in this area do not go straight across, but instead follow the ribs down at an angle. When trying to determine the site of pain, one must follow the rib upward and toward the spine to find the source. This syndrome is also seen in fibromyalgia patients and is a misdiagnosis.

Methods for treatment are local injection of the bilateral joint capsules, which is instantaneous, or an exercise program, which takes longer. Manipulation, or "cracking", of this area should never be done. A range-of-motion exercise program of this area will promote movement without pain and is accomplished by leaning to one side and rotating the dorsal spine, thereby causing the shoulder on that side to go downward and backward. This can be performed at home. Another exercise to add is bending forward completely, arms in, and then bending backwards in similar fashion. If a pain persists a bone scan can be performed as a diagnostic test.

The chest wall pain is sometimes difficult to decipher in that you would always think of heart disease first. But a careful history can determine if true cardiac pain is present. Also cardiac pain will not last for years or result from surgery. I recently examined a woman who had a bypass surgery. The chest pain was present for 4 years. She had a scar from the surgery down the front of the rib cage. She was told that her breasts were too large pulling on the ligament of the mammary glands causing pain. I examined her in a laying down position palpating carefully each costo-cartilage until she and I agreed where the most pain was located. In this instance it was at the 4th costo-cartilage where a scar was located. I injected this area with a steroid and pain killer, and waited the usual "Pannozzo 10 minute test." At 5 minutes the pain was reducing and at 10 minutes the pain of the chest was gone. This is a cure of that source of pain. I have see this type of pain and also pain between ribs, where a muscle strain can occur which may turn into an enthesitis and be painful for awhile. This type of pain when located, and this is the art of medicine and is not easy, then sometimes ultrasound will help along with a certain type of massage I have developed which I call minimobilization. This only works well when the pain source is located precisely.

Fracture of a vertebra in the thoracic spine is very serious for the elderly. It usually follows prolonged sitting, therefore a flexed or bent forward position is assumed for many years in these people. Hip fractures occur in this group also, for the same reason. The loss of calcium or osteoporosis is mainly from inactivity and not a disease state. There is severe pain with this fracture, which can be of any grade, depending on the size of the fracture. The vertebral body can appear wedge-shaped due to the fracture, making the spine angle forward. No extension fractures are seen. The pain however, is from the incidence of fracture to include the body of the vertebra and also the facetal structure. We have discussed this structure before. Remember, the facet or joint is surrounded and held in place by ligamentous tissue which when stretched will be painful. Therefore the pain should be localized to the facet as this is the lingering pain in these patients. There is a pull forward on the joint capsule, causing pain on every movement and turn. The pain can be severe at times. This pain can be treated by reducing the symptoms by local injection of a short acting steroid and a pain killer, but must be done on both sides. Then, the rehab program can commence which consists of extension exercises for range of motion and strength. The surgical approach is to insert a balloon into the body of the vertebra and expand it and fill it with a cement substance to cause rigidity in the body of the vertebra. This is a good procedure, but is less effective when you consider that the facet is not treated. So, for those of you who are suffering from this problem, the above should help you. Seek care from the surgeon if necessary, and a physician who understands the origin of pain and can treat it successfully. Narcotics or other harsh medications are not needed.

Chapter 7
The Lumbar Spine

There are an estimated 50 million people with back pain in the United States alone. My reading of text books and medical books written for the public informs me that the understanding of the causes of pain is not well understood in the medical profession. The usual descriptions of a pain prevail, such as herniated disc, fibromyalgia, lumbar strain, lumbar sprain, and other terms. Physicians have resorted to testing or procedures to determine where a pain originates, but to no appreciable accuracy. For example, anesthesiologists routinely perform injections to *diagnose* facet joint pain, whereas I make a diagnosis from the history and examination and perform facet injections for *treatment* only. A science is present when predictability of result is obtained in treatment for pain. I am disappointed that the medical profession makes up terms to justify the ignorance present in diagnosis and treatment of back pain.

The lumbar spine is constructed in similar fashion to the cervical and thoracic spines. There are 5 lumbar vertebrae, though all are larger than the higher bones as they must support a greater force. The only major conceptual difference between the lumbar vertebrae and the higher vertebrae is the facet joint in the posterior portion, which will be described shortly. The spinal cord extends to the first lumbar vertebra but below that there are only free nerve roots behind the vertebra. These nerve roots travel out of the spine through certain holes, or foramina, and then onward to the area it is to innervate. There is a disc between each vertebra and two facet joints in the posterior portion of the complex, one on each side. The facet joint has a capsule around it, which limits the joint motion and is richly innervated with pain receptors. The facet joints are vertically aligned and are angled about 45° from the sagittal plane, as shown in the picture below. This last fact is important because it determines how the lumbar spine moves, namely forward, backward, and side-to-side, but no rotation.

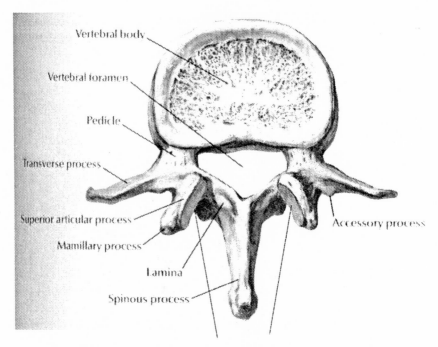

The facet joints are aligned at 45 degrees to the sagittal, or front-back, plane, and 90 degrees on the transverse, or left-right plane. This arrangement will allow forward and backward motion and some side to side motion, but no rotation.

The way I have approached lumbar pain is to determine what the components are of the lumbar spine. There are only five components present as in any other part of the body. I next redefined what a pain is: It is essentially the inability to stretch. You know that is true, especially when you cannot bend forward because of back pain. What occurs when you bend from the waist causing a pain? The thoughts of the last half-century are focused on pressure production in the spine. The old idea is that bending forward causes increased pressure about the disc, which can cause symptoms from the nerves nearby. However, the mechanics of bending seem to have been ignored. When we move any part of our bodies, tissues must stretch to accommodate this motion. If stretch is impossible, then pain is produced as the ligament structure pulls on the bone. This is the basic premise of "mechanical" pain. Over the years of seeing and treating thousands of patients with lumbar pain, without interference of ancillary personnel, who to you are physical therapists and chiropractors, the simple act of bending causing a pain was traced to the joint capsule of the lumbar vertebrae. I began to treat the facet with several means, such as ultrasound to a specific area, and local injection, and mobilization exercises, and began to obtain very good results.

There are basically 6 parameters to examine for low back or lumbar pain. Each movement will bring into play certain structures, and thus can be examined in turn. Slowly, the pain patterns emerged associated with each structure, so the science started to take shape.

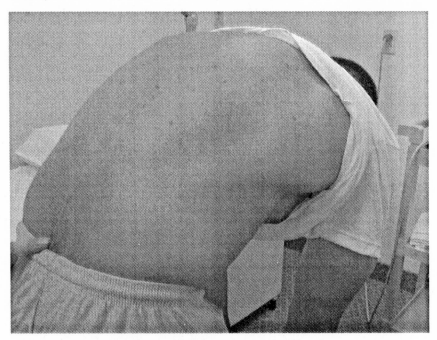

Lumbar flexion, bending forward from the hips.

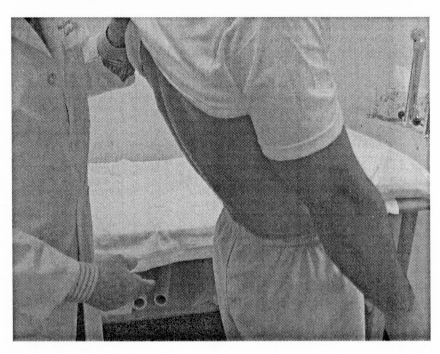

Lumbar extension, bending backward at the hips.

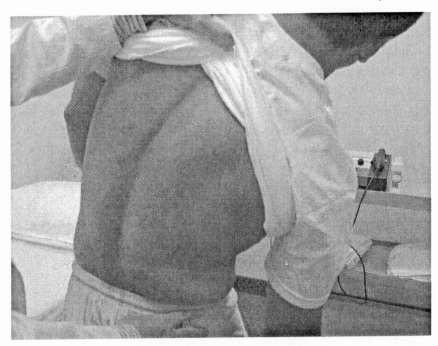

Right lateral bend from the hips.

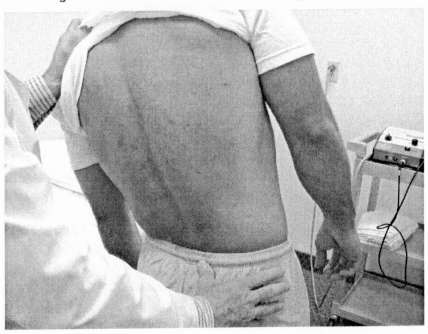

Left lateral bend from the hips.

Next, I had to determine why those structures were painful on examination, and then tie them to x-ray for identification. I had to determine why a pain is lateralized, that is mainly on one side more than the other. I developed a special technique to take x-rays that do show more detail than conventional film to help me make this determination. By cause and effect analysis, I could use this detail to predict which side was the primary and which side was the secondary cause of pain. In other words, I became able to determine which side was the main side to be treated, in spite of the location of the most severe pain to one side. For example, often facet joint pain will be severe on one side, however the motion is restricted mostly on the opposite side, which results in the "swivel effect". The swivel means the restricted side does not move, and excessive motion occurs on the opposite side thus causing pain. The treatment would be to mobilize the restricted side, which is the primary side. It may not be as painful, yet this must be recognized for effective treatment. So even if the most pain was on one side, I could now determine if the pain was a result of another structure based on the physics of motion. When that main side and its structure was located, I then injected a local pain killer to it to determine if I was on the right track. If I could first determine which structure was causing the pain, and then determine which side was the primary, and I could inject it, then this is the best evidence yet of localization of the source of pain tied to a particular motion. The pain killer took ten minutes to take effect. I call this Pannozzo's ten minute test. If I could have the patient repeat the movement on his exam that produced the pain initially, without the pain and with the motion restored, then I have successfully located the source of the pain. This is done without the use of MRI or other special tests. Remember, you cannot diagnose a source of pain using only x-ray or MRI; it is a clinical diagnosis.

I developed a special history tied to the anatomy and physiology of the body, taking into consideration the anatomy of the muscle and ligament structures, their location, and when these structures came into play on an examination. The history of the pattern can be of help in diagnosing the source of the lower extremity pain. If a pain is caused by walking, then it is first a hip joint area pain and not a lower back pain. I have seen many patients limping with a diagnosis of a pinched nerve who have hip joint area pain. These patients are failures in treatment or surgery. Arising from a sitting position is sometimes mistaken for lower back pain or knee pain. This is also hip joint pain.

Next, I developed the examination that we use today which I call *examination by commitment.* By making the patient commit himself to a particular pain to be treated, it ensured both of us that I could now commit myself to treat a particular structure causing pain. This idea has not been done in the past. By this method, the patient and I could determine every source of pain and to categorize the sources of pain as to their importance to be treated in turn. In other words, I simplified the structures down to a primary and a secondary pain source. I formed a pact with the patient to treat a pain which was located by history and physical examination. The follow-up history and examination was done the same way. This obviated the need for questionnaires that you can find in the literature. Identification of the structures causing pain and restoring the normal range of motion of these structures, with the corresponding permanent resolution of pain, is what my practice has been about for 35 years.

There are some basic facts that you should know when experiencing back pain. The first is that when you injure your back, there has to be a change occurring in some structure. This change is tissue damage, as per the accepted definition of pain. There is nothing to the argument that you are getting old, or are experiencing degeneration. There is no "degeneration" and the term should never be used as such. All changes in the bone structure described to you and arthritis, or degeneration, is in reality the body's repair response to injury, which is what the pain is in the first instance. The effect of the injury is to cause pain. Generally pain is worsened with activity, or motion, which requires stretch of tissues to allow the movement. Thus my definition for pain is the inability to stretch, regardless of what the x-ray shows. To describe your back pain in any other way, other than a response to injury, and a structure not being able to stretch because of the injury, is to frighten you, so that you will be overly concerned with your condition.

As mentioned above, if you look at the lumbar spine model and test the movements of the bone structure, it is quite clear that the lumbar vertebrae are not formed to rotate to the side but only to flex or bend forward and backward. The angle of forward looking joints

73

is about 45 degrees. This fact determines the exercise to obtain the normal range of motion. This construction determines that rotational components are not present here, only bending forward or backward, and this is easily shown. Any manipulation or forced rotation causing a "pop" should never be done. Knowing the normal physiology of the spine determines what weight bearing the spine can do. One of our proprietary exercises is to bend forward and to the left or right at 45 degrees to mobilize the facet joint. This is done by keeping the knees straight and touching or attempting to touch the palm to its corresponding shin bone on each side. The old Williams flexion exercises are outmoded.

So first, if you cannot bend while standing, then the pain is from the back of the vertebrae. The axis of motion is in front of the facet joints, therefore the joint capsule must stretch to allow this motion, and the disc must compress. While most focus on the disc and its pressure change, I focus on the facet joint capsule. By careful examination a tender area will be noted that is over the facet joint. There are other areas that may be somewhat tender, but pressure over the proper joint will produce the worst pain. The facet capsule has been demonstrated to be the pain generator of the facet joint complex in several studies. However the old idea of the facet synovium being the culprit still persists in many physicians, who therefore think bending backwards is the way to stress facet joints. This is the reason they perform injections for their diagnosis and I diagnose by examination. For the reader, if there is pain produced only with bending forward, you can be assured this is a non-surgical condition, and MRIs, epidurals, manipulation, or physical therapy are not necessary.

If your pain occurs mostly when bending forward, then the treatment that you can do at home is to stand with your feet spread past your shoulders, and to bend first to the left, then to the right, with your knees straight and stiff. If you can do this simple maneuver and take aspirin, most of your pain will disappear in several hours, because you have repositioned your vertebrae for normal function. This is not simplistic. This actually works well.

Secondly if your pain is produced by bending backwards, then the annulus or disc ligament is injured, and the treatment is different. Bending backward necessitates that the annulus must stretch somewhat to allow this motion. When the annulus cannot stretch well, it pulls on the vertebral body to which it is attached, thus causing the deep pain that people feel with this motion. Now the main side is determined as the primary source of pain, thus naming the secondary side also. The structure is located by pain pattern and clinical examination, and then a film is taken to help with the treatment approach to discover why the structure is painful. I inject the outer annulus at the bony insertion and patients bend backwards without pain immediately afterward. This procedure is my own, and it is not yet taught in schools. It is the end result of a long and intricate study of spine mechanics. Sometimes ultrasound alone can be a very effective treatment, along with specific exercise for the annular structure. The exercise to do is to bend backwards, increasing the range each time and to hold the backward stretch for 6 seconds, ten times, which is one minute, three or four times in a day. Aspirin is again the drug of choice, although if the pain is severe enough, oral steroids such as prednisone can be taken for a few days.

Usually I hear that a pain in the leg or buttock, or calf must be a "pinched nerve." This is far from reality, in that there are several structures that can produce lower extremity pain. The L_5-S_1 facet joint can produce pain into the buttock. The L_{4-5} facet will produce buttock pain to the side of the buttock and lower down into the side of the thigh. The annulus at L_{4-5} level will produce pain or aching or tingling sensation to the side of the calf. An L_5 nerve lesion usually will cause a tingling in the large toe and weakness of the foot dorsiflexors. An S_1 radiculopathy will cause a tingling down the thigh and calf and into the small toe. A nerve lesion, or radiculopathy, can be diagnosed by electromyogram at 2-3 weeks after the onset of pain or weakness. Higher levels of lumbar pain sources are similarly located by history and clinical examination. The L_{3-4} level will produce pain in the anterior lateral thigh or upper leg. The structure again is a joint if the pain is produced by bending forward or the annulus if the pain is produced by bending backwards. The source of the pain is determined clinically and then the film is taken and analyzed to produce an accurate exercise program. A little known pain syndrome causing a tingle like sensation to the side of the calf can come from a pulled muscle at the distal or lower thigh adductor muscles, and if suspected, can be found by palpation. This is a very important source of lower extremity pain.

If rapid recovery is needed by the patient or the pain is too severe, then we can inject the offending structure, which will decrease the pain in 10 minutes therefore restoring the normal range of motion. This relief of pain this quickly becomes a permanent relief of pain in 10 to 12 hours. This is routine treatment in my office. This is not available to your physicians unless they are trained in these techniques. Epidural injections are not recommended because this procedure is not aimed at any particular structure causing pain. Indeed, if your physician knows where the pain source is, then why not treat that source? MRI cannot tell where the source of pain is located because it is a static test, in the lying down position, done by someone who has not taken a history or examined you. This is a severe burden on the radiologist. Similarly, if a physical therapist or chiropractor is given the freedom to diagnose your condition, the chance of a good outcome is very low.

My experience in treating 12,000 patients with low back pain shows that the average number of treatments per patient is 4, and the satisfaction is 97% by questionnaire and or examination. Our back to work studies done several years apart show that patients who are injured at work, go back to their same job without time off or retraining 91% of the time. The remaining patients who did not return to work were frauds or retired. This is true and these studies were done 5 years apart using consecutive patients, not selected for this study except an injury at work.

Be extremely careful when taking physical therapy treatments for back pain which are not remotely related to lumbar structures, such as treadmill, swimming or other aquatic treatments. Knowing these facts, it is plainly seen that water therapy is not the treatment of choice. Also be wary of manipulation because this is another form of injury to the lumbar structures.

Another entity that we have researched and treat is the lumbo-sacral list. We actually have written the only article on the diagnosis and effective treatment of this condition. A list is a sideways bend of the spine due to injury. This can be very dramatic at times, and you will notice someone listing will literally be bent over to the side due to pain. The hallmark of the list is the absolute inability to bend toward the opposite side of the list. For example, if a person is bent to the right, they will not be able to bend left at all when standing upright. This entity is the result of an extreme facet injury usually from a lifting injury. The list is not a disc injury of any kind. We have found that lifting an object from an angle tends to bend the spine and can hurt the facet on the opposite side. We inject the facets at the problem level and this predictably improves in three treatment days. The key to the treatment is the facet joints. Listing is not from a muscle imbalance or muscle injury and does not need muscle relaxers or electrical stimulation. It absolutely does not require surgery. Manipulation will not help this and I have seen a few cases where it actually worsened the patient. Ultrasound may be helpful as it improves the stretchability of the joint capsules and offers a pain relieving effect. The picture below is of a woman who came to see me two weeks after injuring her back. She was bent to the right, and unable to bend to the left. The film on the left was taken the day she came, and the bend to the right is quite obvious. We treated her facet joints at the L_{4-5} level and the next day her curve was improved, as you can see by the film on the right. She was able to bend to the left when asked, and her spine continued to straighten over the next two days. This treatment is predictable and effective.

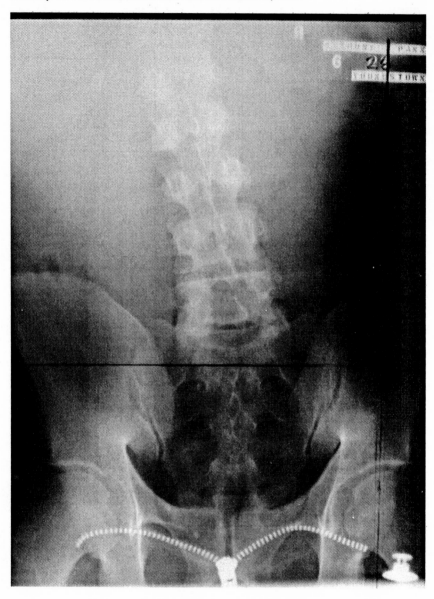

Listing patient before treatment

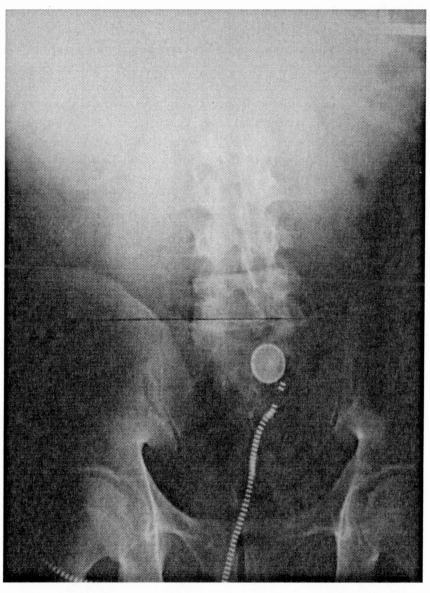

Listing patient after treatment, two days later.

The sacroiliac joint has been mentioned often as a source for low back and buttock pain that may even refer down the thigh. This joint is between the sacrum and ilium, two bones that help comprise the pelvis. This is the most stable joint in the body, made very strong by the thick ligament connectors between the two bones. I have seen many cases where a person was in a bad car wreck or had a fall from an elevated area and had pelvis fractures but yet the joint was intact. This joint had better be strong, for it must transmit all the force from the spine horizontally and then down toward the hip. See the picture below.

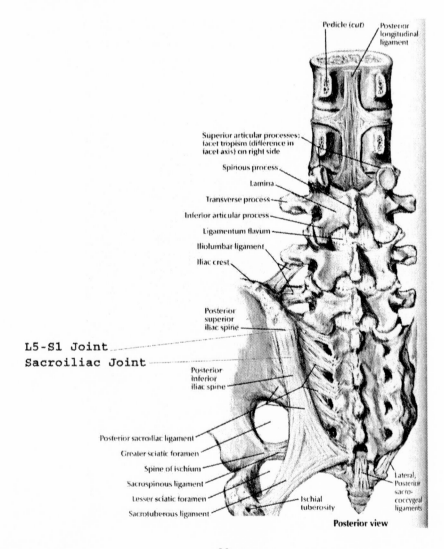

Posterior view

Before the 1920's the medical community felt that all back pain was from the sacroiliac joint, not from the disc or facet joint. After some observations of herniated discs in cadavers, the focus changed away from the SIJ and to structures in the back itself. Over the past fifteen years or so the diagnosis of sacroiliac joint syndrome has seen resurgence as physicians were having a large amount of patients who were not improving from the typical treatments or had symptoms and examination findings that did not fit the "accepted" diagnoses. A significant number of physicians are now injecting the sacroiliac joints again.

There have been many studies performed over the years looking at the SI joint which show that this cannot be a pain producing structure. The motion of the SI joint is extremely limited, only a few degrees or so. It is not made to move any more than this. If this joint was mobile, our spines would not have a base of support and we would never be walking upright. Some doctors state that the SI joint develops "ridges" and other arthritic changes as we age, however years ago when these "ridges" were investigated they were found to be covered with cartilage, indicating that these ridges are actually adaptive, meant to make the SI joint even more strong and stable as they interlock. Any severe "arthritic" change in any other joint has no cartilage covering. This is an extremely significant finding about the SI joint. The most basic contradiction with the idea that the SI joint is the cause of back pain concerns motion. The other physicians will say that the SI joint developed the arthritic changes because of motion, yet the joint does not allow movement, and in fact gets less mobile as we age.

As shown in the picture above, the L_5-S_1 facet joint is very close to the SI joint, as are the iliolumbar ligaments. The hip joint is very close as well, just to the outside of the SI joint. These are structures that must allow motion and be stretchable. I would recommend that you do not include the sacroiliac joint as a cause of your pain. Instead look to an abnormality with these other structures inhibiting their ability to move.

Some patients have come into my office with lower back pain, and they stated that their physician told them the pain was from osteoporosis. Osteoporosis is a weakening of the bone from decreased activity and hormonal changes that can occur as we age. Post-menopausal women are most susceptible for the condition, but men and women alike can get this from inactivity. The bone architecture is normal in osteoporosis, there is just less of it. The bone is weaker and has greater chance of developing a fracture, often at the hip, wrist, or thoracic or lumbar spines. When a vertebra fractures from osteoporosis it compresses and will be wedge-shaped in the front.

New vertebral fractures can be very painful, and this should always be a consideration in someone with this diagnosis. However, the majority of lumbar vertebral compression fractures have been asymptomatic in my experience, meaning that the bone fractured prior to their visit to me. If a fracture develops slowly and the vertebral body compresses slowly, it may not be painful, and the fracture will be found on an x-ray. The person will develop pain from the facet joint though, because the wedging of the vertebra causes the facet joint capsule to be continually stretched, which results in pain. I have found that I have helped people greatly by treating the facet joints even though they have a documented thoracic or lumbar compression fracture. An extension exercise program should be included with the facet joint treatment. The idea I want you to know is that compression fractures are not always painful, and the facet joints may be the major component of the pain problem from osteoporotic compression fractures.

Of course the details of the more complex pain syndromes cannot be described here, but the message you should be receiving here is that back pain can be completely understood and treated successfully. I have read other texts in preparation for this book, and I have been disappointed in the information that the lay person can find. Most of the authors conclude that back pain is not understood, and have recommended alternative treatments. My advice to you is to ignore alternative methods and to stick to the science that is already established, as I have described it above. The outcome instruments in the literature are based on scales such as the visual analog scale or SF36, or the Roland scale and others. The problem with these scales is that the questions asked are a mishmash of symptomology not based on anatomy and physiology of motion or weight bearing and include several anatomical sites of pain, therefore nullifying the answers. So, to repeat, a normal range of motion of the lower back indicates a normal back, period. The idea of a chronic pain which is untreatable and therefore disabling is not true. We must get a handle on this problem. This is my solution and should work for you and your doctor.

As far as treatments are concerned, early on if the pain is not severe, then an exercise program is prescribed based on the film taken, and an anti-inflammatory medication is given along with ultra sound heat. If the patient is elderly, then a pelvic traction can be added. If the pain is impacting either work or play, or routine chores, then the local injections can be added for the facet or joint pain of forward bending, or annular injection given for pain of extension or bending backward. Sometimes a combination of facetal and annular injection is necessary and is easily accomplished. In any case, the treatment is on target as to structure, and the result is predictable, and is a science. Testing is usually not necessary such as MRI, and CT scan. If the same pain persists over one week, then these tests are to be done. The bone scan is the best screening test in my opinion. Our statistics over several years shows that we have treated 12.000 patients and the average treatment time is 4 days of treatment. No more that 2-3 patients were referred for surgery in this series.

Sample Case

A 43 year-old male came about 150 miles to see me, bypassing some large and respected pain centers. He had back pain for roughly 4 years, and over the years he was given treatments like bicycle and swimming. X-Rays and MRIs were ordered, and he underwent laminectomy with no help. He was taking narcotic analgesics for relief. On examination his pain was traced to the L_{4-5} and L_5-S_1 levels, where the surgical scar was most pronounced. These levels were mobilized over 5 visits with injection and ultrasound modality. His pain resolved completely with our treatment. We know this is true because he returned 8 months later after hurting his back is a work injury and he stated he was doing well without pain in that interval. Back pain can be treated effectively with the concept of mobilization and direct, specific treatments.

Chapter 8
Hip pain

The most often misdiagnosed pain syndrome is hip pain, which many times is mistaken for low back pain. The obvious difference is that the hip is involved in dynamic weight bearing, walking or in other words transferring the weight of the body from one position to another. The lumbar spine is involved generally in static weight bearing, or standing, whereas the hip is involved in movement of the body to another position such as climbing steps, arising from a chair or getting out of bed. Limping is also a hip manifestation and not lumbar in origin.

The pelvis forms the socket of the hip joint and the femur, or thigh bone, meets the socket forming the hip joint. The front of the hip joint has a very strong capsule which limits backward motion. When we stand in place, we actually do not use any muscles to keep ourselves upright, but this ligament is so strong it supports our hip. The back of the capsule is more lax to allow us to flex the hip, which raises the knee into the air. There are a few important muscles that move our hip which could be causes of pain. The hip flexor muscle starts at the back and attaches to the thigh bone near the hip joint, and it allows us raise our knee into the air. The external rotator muscles are along the back of the hip and allow us to turn our foot outward. The adductor muscles begin on the pelvis close to the hip joint and continue down the inside of the thigh. See the pictures below.

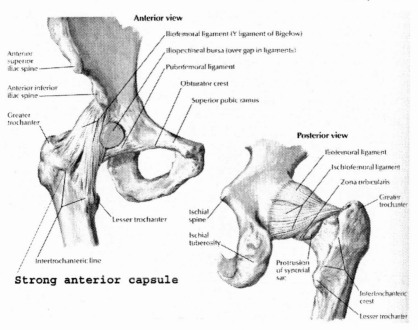

Anterior view

Iliofemoral ligament (Y ligament of Bigelow)

Iliopectineal bursa (over gap in ligaments)

Pubofemoral ligament

Obturator crest

Superior pubic ramus

Anterior superior iliac spine

Anterior inferior iliac spine

Greater trochanter

Lesser trochanter

Intertrochanteric line

Strong anterior capsule

Posterior view

Iliofemoral ligament

Ischiofemoral ligament

Zona orbicularis

Greater trochanter

Ischial spine

Ischial tuberosity

Protrusion of synovial sac

Intertrochanteric crest

Lesser trochanter

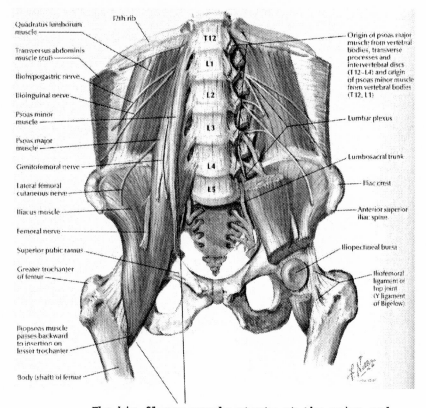

The hip flexor muscle starts at the spine and attaches to the lesser trochanter. This muscle allows us to raise our knees into the air.

The hip has a unique examination based on its design and function. The function of the hip joint is to rotate in its connection with the pelvis. I have developed a simple examination for this joint, which is done in a sitting position. The examiner holds the knee with one hand and the ankle with the other hand to rotate the ankle-that is hip joint by rotating the ankle up towards the other leg, and recording the degree motion with or without pain. Likewise the opposite motion is recorded by moving the ankle away from the other leg. The hip flexor tendon is then tested by having the patient raise the knee and keep the knee elevated against resistance. The hips are then compared for pain and motion. If the pain occurs on external rotation, then the pain is located to the medial hip capsule. If the pain occurs on internal rotation, then the pain occurs in the lateral hip capsule. If the patient cannot keep the knee elevated, there is a hip flexor tendonitis. Rarely are both hips painful at the same time or intensity or show a decreased motion. As you recall, all joints have a normal range of motion. When a joint capsule is painful, then the normal range of motion is decreased because it hurts to move it. See pictures below.

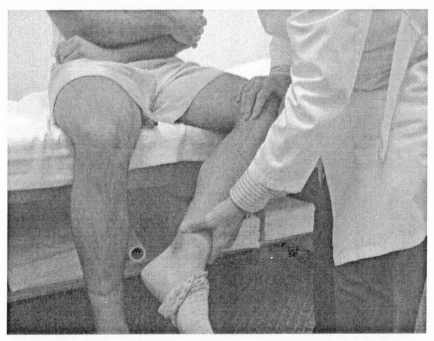

Testing external rotation of the hip by rotating the foot toward the other. The medial capsule is assessed with this maneuver. Testing the lateral capsule is performed by rotating the foot in the opposite direction.

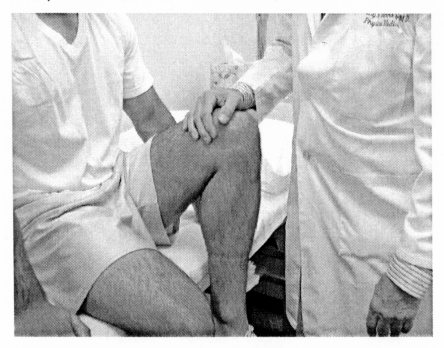

Testing the hip flexor by having the patient
raise the knee and maintain this position
against downward pressure.

If the lumbar range of motion is normal without pain, and the
hip capsule is painful, then no lumbar pain is present and the hip
is treated. Sometimes hip pain and lumbar pain are present at the
same time. Then the decision as to which is treated first is posed to
the patient. He or she will decide which pain is worse and should be
treated first. Later, the other can be treated.

The structures of the hip have certain pain patterns if injured.
In my experience, the hip flexor tendon is commonly painful. Pain
from this can be in the front of the hip or in back of it, and will be
painful when getting out of a chair. The external rotator tendon can
be painful, which will cause pain in the back of the hip. This can be
painful in two areas, where the muscle starts in the back of the hip
near the sacrum and toward the side, where the muscle attaches
on the back of the thigh bone. The adductor origin is an important
cause of groin pain. The hip capsule can be painful in the front,
or inside or medial capsule, or lateral or posterior. Walking pain

and thigh pain are usually related to the lateral and postero-lateral capsule. Sitting pain is often medial hip capsule in origin. It is very interesting that the description of President Kennedy having sitting pain was missed as hip in origin because the low back was always treated. Who knows if history could have been different if he was not medicated so heavily for it. Turning over in bed is hip pain also.

The hip will refer pain into the thigh, but the adductor muscle needs to be evaluated for this symptom too. The adductor muscle begins near the hip joint and travels down the inside of the thigh attaching broadly to the bone from the knee all the way up toward the hip. A pull-type injury to the muscle attachment will cause pain in the thigh, which may also refer to the calf. Often when asked where the pain begins the patient will put their hand on the front or outside of the mid-thigh. This is a sure sign of adductor pain. If the inside of the thigh is palpated just opposite of where they feel the pain starts, a very tender area is usually found, which is the best method to diagnose this problem. I routinely inject the area of maximum tenderness and the symptoms resolve.

The hip may also refer pain toward the knee, especially the inside portion. It is a well known referral pattern, but unfortunately more than a few people have had knee replacements when they should have had their hip treated! The hip can cause true knee pain as well because of the way the hip affects the knee. If the hip capsule does not allow normal motion, then abnormal motion will occur at the hip and at the knee. This is especially true if there is a hip flexion contracture which will force the knee into a bent position. All abnormal motions on the thigh bone will actually be magnified because of the distance from the hip.

X-rays and/or MRI for diagnosis of hip pain as a pre-operative step is not a good idea. In my experience, x-ray can be a help for a diagnosis. It can show why the hip is painful, usually from a leg length difference. I have seen patients with the worst looking x-rays walk almost normal, however.

Any aspect of hip pain can be treated by exercise, or if severe enough with a decreased range of motion, an injection of a steroid. An injection can bring marvelous results overnight, which is my experience. Ultrasound is an excellent choice also because it offers a deep heat, which cannot be obtained from hot packs. The heat allows the capsule to soften and stretch and is useful in my opinion.

There are specific exercises that we give to patients to mobilize the hip capsule when necessary. The medial hip capsule can be painful with sitting and can refer pain behind it into the buttock. The medial hip capsule is stretched by spreading the feet beyond shoulder's width and then leaning to the opposite site, in an exaggerated groin stretch. If there is a hip flexion contracture, the hip will be bent and unable to straighten out to its normal position. This may not be painful at the hip, but the front of the knee will be painful because the front of the knee will be stretched constantly to compensate for the hip. The front of the hip is stretched two possible ways, either lying on your stomach on the bed, or leaning the chest against the wall with the foot on the contracted side behind the buttock. See the picture below.

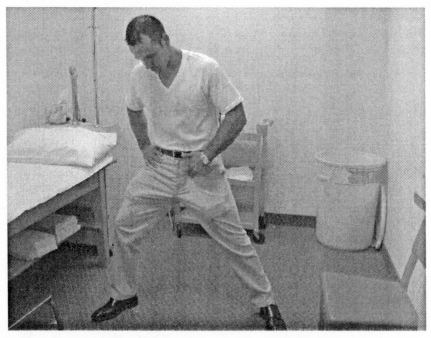

The left medial hip is stretched by leaning to the right in an exaggerated groin stretch. This should be felt in the inside of the left hip where the model is pointing.

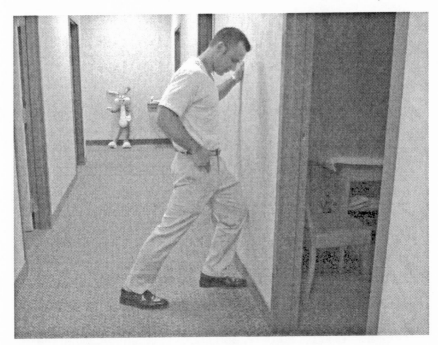

This is a picture of an exercise for a right
hip flexion contracture. The right foot is
behind the buttock, which stretches the front
of the hip. This should be felt in the front
of the hip where the model is pointing.

So to recap, if your pain is present while walking it is hip in origin
and not low back. Sitting pain may also be hip in origin. Low back
pain in contrast will occur when standing and bending.

Let me take a moment to remind you that pain syndromes are
well understood. There is no reason to have pain more than a few
days if the diagnosis and treatment is correct. No need exists for
medication stronger that aspirin or its derivatives. No narcotics are
ever needed, and loss of work is not necessary. Sick behavior is to
be avoided by the patient for their own good. If you are not getting
better in a few days, then my advice to you as a physician and a
patient is to move on until you find someone who knows about pain
syndromes.

Chapter 9
Knee Pain

The knee joint is as we all know is usually injured in sports and is a major pain source of pain in the elderly. It is subject of surgery, bracing, arthroscopic surgery, and knee replacement. What makes up the knee joint? Why does it require so much management and produce so much pain? I will attempt to explain it to you.

Anatomically, the knee joint joins the femur to the tibia. Outside of the joint itself, there is a complex ligament structure that not only binds the bones together, but as all ligaments, allows normal motion and also prevents excessive motion. When the normal motion allowed is exceeded, pain then occurs. The complex ligament allows the bones that it binds to rotate in and out, and to flex or bend, and to straighten out. Fibers in the ligament or capsule of the knee are arranged in layers with the orientation of the fibers as the picture shows.

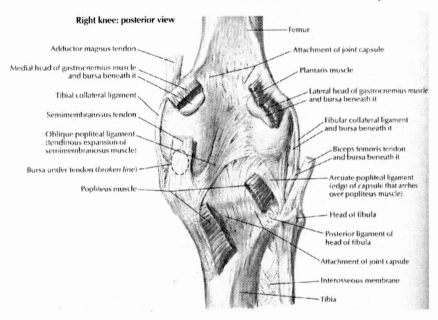

Right knee: posterior view

Adductor magnus tendon

Medial head of gastrocnemius muscle and bursa beneath it

Tibial collateral ligament

Semimembranosus tendon

Oblique popliteal ligament (tendinous expansion of semimembranosus muscle)

Bursa under tendon (broken line)

Popliteus muscle

Femur

Attachment of joint capsule

Plantaris muscle

Lateral head of gastrocnemius muscle and bursa beneath it

Fibular collateral ligament and bursa beneath it

Biceps femoris tendon and bursa beneath it

Arcuate popliteal ligament (edge of capsule that arches over popliteus muscle)

Head of fibula

Posterior ligament of head of fibula

Attachment of joint capsule

Interosseous membrane

Tibia

Attached to the knee joint capsule is the cartilage, which we know as the menisci. There is a lateral and a medial meniscus. These cartilages are attached to the capsule on the outer perimeter of the tibia as the picture shows. These cartilages are flat to allow the femur to rotate on when and you use your knee. This action is necessary in the design of the joint to give you full seamless use of the joint when walking and running and climbing and the other many uses in every day life and in sports. The meniscus is flat, so the chance of injuring or tearing it is extremely remote. In addition there are two ligaments that prevent excessive front and back motion of the tibia on the femur known as the anterior and posterior cruciate ligaments.

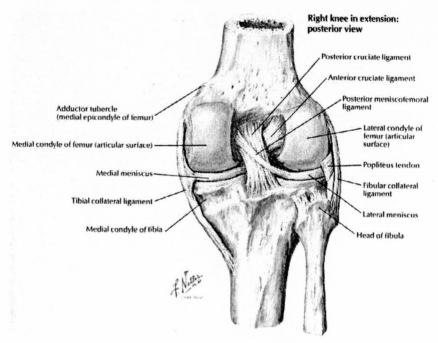

Right knee in extension: posterior view

Posterior cruciate ligament

Anterior cruciate ligament

Posterior meniscofemoral ligament

Adductor tubercle (medial epicondyle of femur)

Lateral condyle of femur (articular surface)

Medial condyle of femur (articular surface)

Popliteus tendon

Medial meniscus

Fibular collateral ligament

Tibial collateral ligament

Lateral meniscus

Medial condyle of tibia

Head of fibula

Surrounding the inside of the knee joint is a lining called the knee synovium. This sensitive tissue serves to lubricate the inside of the knee, and it also is the source of fluid that we know as "water on the knee". This fluid can mean a disease state, but most of time means that the joint was injured.

None of the structures above will move the knee tibia or femur. This function is done by the patellar tendon and quadriceps muscle in front of the knee connecting to the tibia, which allows you to kick. The flexion or bending of the knee is accomplished by the flexor tendons attached to the muscles of the back of the thigh. There are basically two, one along the back of the outer part of the tibia and one along the inside of the tibia. There are then, three groups of muscles that control the knee movement.

Functionally, the knee bears weight in a 180 degree extension mode normally. This allows you to stand on one leg, without difficulty. Anything less than 180 degrees is a knee flexion contracture and will lead to an abnormal function. If the knee must work at less than straight or 180 degrees, the most weight bearing will occur in the front of the knee joint. The capsule of the knee allows a certain amount of rotation of the tibia on the femur when walking and turning a corner, and changing direction when walking or running.

The hip joint has a major effect on the function of the knee joint. Remember our previous discussion of the physiology of weight bearing. The knee pain must be viewed as an abnormal usage of the joint, especially in the non-athletic population, although all knee pain has trauma in the history. If the hip does not function as designed, in other words has a restricted motion, then the hip will place the knee in an abnormal position to work or function. For example, if the hip cannot externally rotate in walking, having a medial hip joint capsule restriction, the knee will be painful at the posterior medial part. If the hip cannot adequately internally rotate in walking having a lateral hip contracture, then the pain will occur at the posterior lateral part of the knee and lateral knee area. If the hip has a flexion contracture, then the knee will be forced to have a flexion contracture, which leads to abnormal weight bearing at the front of the knee joint with puffiness and pain.

The hip component description above came from a research project that was outlined when I had a medical student for rotation in my office for 3 weeks, on two separate occasions. The research was first done by charting the knee problems and hip problems on the same patient. The next rotation entailed a protocol to predict what the hip would show when the knee was charted by exam. The treatment of any knee pain then follows this protocol in my practice. So always have the hip evaluated first before any type of surgery or treatment is tried. If your hip is painful, treat it before the knee is treated.

When examining the knee for pain, the lack of certain motions will give you the cause of the pain if the physiology of the knee is known and is taken into consideration. The knee must be able to reach full extension. To test for a knee flexion contracture, have the person sit on the examination table and straighten the knee. If the knee cannot straighten to 180° then there is a contracture and the back of the joint must be mobilized. See the picture below.

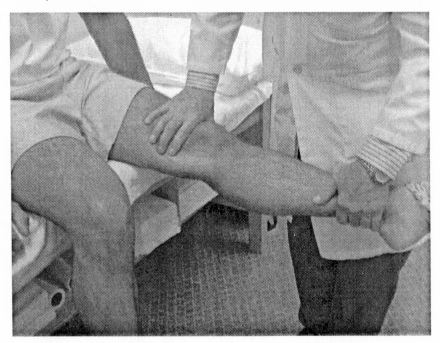

Testing for a knee flexion contracture by extending the knee.

The other knee ligaments are assessed by various examination maneuvers designed to stress them. You will probably remember how the doctor moved your leg to the right and left or pulled on your leg like he was opening a desk drawer. These are all tests to evaluate ligaments.

The other structure to be examined is the patella and patellar tendon in front of the knee. This is the attachment of the quadriceps muscle to the tibia to give you the ability to kick your leg. The patella should be freely movable without pain on compression. See the picture below.

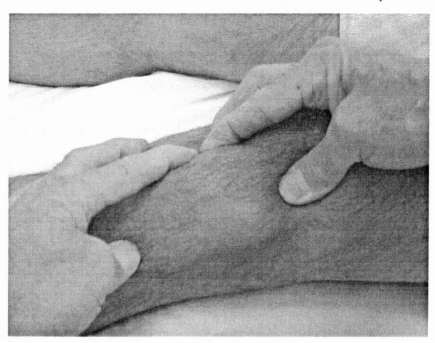

In addition, in the back of the knee there is the flexor tendon of the knee at the medial and lateral parts of the tibia which gives us the ability to bend our knees. These tendon attachments can be tender and painful, but are easily treated by ultrasound and stretching, or mobilization, or by local injection which is a sure cure. The capsule is a source of knee pain, and so is the meniscus attached to it. The articular cartilage, which is the cartilage attached to the ends of the bones, can be a pain source as well though I believe this is secondary to the capsule. The capsule attaches to the bone in that area, so that the injury to the ligament nearby will produce calcium formation as a repair process and will involve the cartilage.

Rarely do I see a total exam of the knee in a report, except in my office. All structures must be palpated, and charted as to precisely where the pain is located in the knee or around the knee joint.

All imaging studies should be performed in the weight bearing position. The pelvic obliquity or short limb must be analyzed as a possible cause of abnormal weight bearing thus causing some of the trauma of the knee. In my office patients with knee pain have x-rays in the standing position—the weight bearing position—the physiological position. MRIs are now able to be performed upright, which is ultimately offers much more valuable information that the typical study performed lying down.

The common knee pain syndromes are easily explained if the proper physiology is known. It is only a matter of reasoning to figure out the cause of any particular symptom. If weight bearing is shifted to the front of the knee because of a hip flexion contracture or knee flexion contracture, the front of the knee will become painful over time. The joint capsule or ligaments that hold the femur and tibia bones together will be stretched and will become swollen and painful. This syndrome is called the Anterior Knee Capsulitis. This is absolutely not a surgical condition. This is treated by stretching the back of the knee joint or capsule. This can be accomplished by using ultrasound followed by mobilization exercises. Usually the posterior medial knee capsule is tight or scarred down by repeated injuries or excessive sitting. This is why this problem is found primarily in the elderly. It is also associated with a flexion contracture of the hip, which will not allow the full extension of the hip and knee. This is why this is found in the elderly because of excessive sitting.

The medial meniscus is attached to the medial collateral ligament. If there is an abnormal weight bearing at the medial part of the knee, it is possible to have a meniscus tear. But remember, the capsule of the knee protects this structure and must be torn out before the meniscus can be damaged. The narrowing of the medial meniscus is said to be because it is worn out. This is absolutely the wrong thinking. The cartilage will narrow if squeezed by the capsule developing a contracture. Removing a cartilage because it is narrow and torn is not good thinking. One should mobilize the medial compartment of the knee, and the cartilage will function normally. We are doing original research on the problem in my office at this time.

Anterior Cruciate Ligament tear, although a commonly made diagnosis, is an extremely difficult injury to have. Looking at a model of the knee with intact ligament structures does not lend itself to injury easily, because of the capsule that holds the knee together must be ripped out completely to get at this ligament. The same idea holds true for the posterior cruciate ligament. In other words, there are other structures protecting these ligaments, but the surgeons do not mention them. I rarely see a detailed examination of the knee by the physician, but see MRI which in my experience cannot accurately show these structures. I also see "evaluations" by the physical therapist and then their treatments, but without the surgeon directly involved. I do hands on treatments, and the technicians are to help me.

To treat the knee successfully, one must know about and be able to distinguish each and every structure outlined above. The normal anatomy of the knee for treatment purposes is divided into the inside of the knee and the outside of the knee. The outside of the knee contains primarily the joint capsule which is a ligament that binds the femur and tibia together completely around the joint. In general, ligaments are the most painful areas of the knee, but are the least taken into consideration because there is essentially no surgery for capsulitis. The hip is always treated to normal range of motion before the knee is treated. Dr Grelsamer in his book on the knee is absolutely correct when he and I agree that if the physician does not examine the knee, but orders tests and refers you to a therapist without control, then walk away from that physician.

Each side of the knee joint can be isolated as being painful that is, front, back and medial side and lateral side. One can determine if the pain is internal to the knee or external to the knee joint, or capsule. If heat is present of a moderate degree or cool to touch, then the capsule is involved solely. If there is more than a moderate degree of heat with redness and possible fluid, then the problem is internal to the knee and is an indication of a synovitis, a more serious problem requiring a more extensive workup.

In the area of treatment, it is important to disregard the notion of weakness, and to know that the back of the knee must fully extend to produce a normal range of motion of the knee to get relief of pain. Our knee exercises are based on quad exercises to stretch the posterior capsule, not for strength. The knee cap malalignment is based on the hip function, and is not an entity in itself. You can have scarring of the retinaculum around the knee cap to prevent the normal excursion of the patella, and this is easily found on examination. The treatment for this is to mobilize the tight area. If it is related to the hip, then the hip must be treated to a normal range of motion. Other locations of pain around the knee can include the distal thigh muscles—a pulled muscle or tendon insertion about the knee area from the knee flexors of the thigh. These areas are treated locally by the physician.

Steroids can be used successfully in the treatment of the capsule and ligaments of the knee and tendons that move the knee. It is also useful in treating inflammation of the synovium if temporarily inflamed. The literature supporting the idea of only three injections into the joint per year is based on an observation of someone when he saw a knee that was injected many times. He erroneously attributed the changes to the steroid treatment. I read those articles, and the science was missing. First, the reason the injections were given was not discussed. The disease process was not found to prompt the injections. In my reading of the literature, I surmised that the knee changes were based on a capsulitis and not in the knee itself, where the shots were placed. The knee just was not treated, period. This is important because many operations have taken place because the capsules were not treated with ant-inflammatory drugs for a cure. We use only short acting steroids with a working time of approximately 4 hours. The reason that good results are obtained is because the structure causing the problem was successfully found and treated.

I have treated from 1996 over a thousand knees with good success, without surgical interference. Now, some of the knees that I see are so bad that knee replacement surgery can be the most efficient way to give a patient relief of his pain. In regard to arthroscopic surgery, the lavage procedure has been discredited in the New England Journal of Medicine two years ago. They do not feel the idea of trimming the cartilage is a good physiologic solution for knee pain. Remember, most knee pain is caused by the ligament surrounding the knee which connects the femur to the tibia and also connects to the meniscus. This is the area of excessive bone growth following a knee injury, not on the inside of the knee. Is the calcium formation a disease? Decidedly not! This is merely a response to injury to the ligament bone connection, and should not be removed because more scar formation will take place and perhaps be more painful than before. No, an accurate evaluation by a physician will treat the underlying problem that produced the bone spur.

There are many terms used to describe painful knees. You should know what is meant by these terms, and if they are diagnostic in their meaning. <u>Osteoarthritis</u> is an imprecise diagnosis. In my experience with thousands of patients, there is usually trauma in the history. These knees on x-ray will show narrowing of a medial compartment usually, but narrowing can also be found in the lateral compartment. A good history will always elicit trauma. Degenerative joint disease is also not precise as a diagnosis. This is another term for trauma. <u>Osteoporosis</u> is an x-ray diagnosis primarily. There is an index by agreement that if the level of calcium falls below an arbitrary number, then this can be your diagnosis. By itself, this diagnosis is not treatable as a knee pain. This shows in the elderly who sit a lot. The pain is still from other structures of the knee and requires close examination, not testing. <u>Chondromalacia</u> is an imprecise diagnosis, merely meaning excessive wear under the patella. If one walks with the knee bent, then the weight of the body will be borne on the underside of the patella. The treatment of this problem is to document the flexion contracture and then to mobilize the back of the knee joint capsule, thereby restoring the normal weight bearing of the knee as it was designed.

I remember a particular incident when I volunteered to be a sideline physician for our high school football games on Friday night. A young man injured his left knee during play, which I examined on the field. I determined that there was a capsular sprain present and was easily treated. The next day this young man came in to the office with his father. The father explained how he had injured his knee when he played football in high school and then had an operation on his knee, and it was still a painful "football knee." He asked me about whirlpool to treat the boy's knee. I explained that the water does not treat the cause of the pain and that the newer methods would do just fine. He immediately took his son out of my office to the YMCA where he could get water therapy. I did not see this patient for 4 years until he came to the office on his own. By that time he had had both knees operated, and was in pain daily with a scar on both knees. This is part of the lore of knee injury in sports.

Chapter 10
Ankle, Foot, and Heel Pain

The ankle and foot are the last weight bearing organs of the body. The ankle will bear weight or otherwise function where the hip and knee places it to work. The ankle is made up of several smaller bones, called the tarsal bones, which are analogous to the wrist bones. The normal weight bearing surface of the ankle joint, or ankle mortise, is the bone structure made up of the distal parts of the calf bones, the tibia and fibula, and the first small ankle bone, the talus. The tibia and fibula surround the talus to provide stability to the ankle. The rest of the tarsal bones are connected and the whole thing is bound together with connective tissue. See picture below.

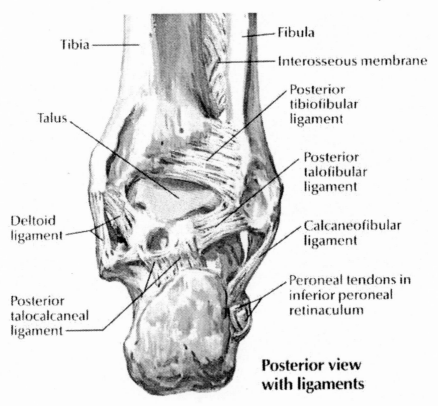

Tibia

Talus

Deltoid
ligament

Posterior
talocalcaneal
ligament

Fibula

Interosseous membrane

Posterior
tibiofibular
ligament

Posterior
talofibular
ligament

Calcaneofibular
ligament

Peroneal tendons in
inferior peroneal
retinaculum

**Posterior view
with ligaments**

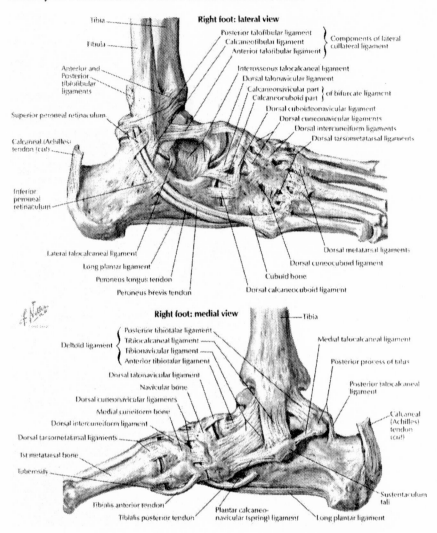

Right foot: lateral view

Tibia
Fibula
Anterior and Posterior tibiofibular ligaments
Superior peroneal retinaculum
Calcaneal (Achilles) tendon (cut)
Inferior peroneal retinaculum
Lateral talocalcaneal ligament
Long plantar ligament
Peroneus longus tendon
Peroneus brevis tendon

Posterior talofibular ligament
Calcaneofibular ligament } Components of lateral collateral ligament
Anterior talofibular ligament
Interosseous talocalcaneal ligament
Dorsal talonavicular ligament
Calcaneonavicular part } of bifurcate ligament
Calcaneocuboid part
Dorsal cuboideonavicular ligament
Dorsal cuneonavicular ligament
Dorsal intercuneiform ligaments
Dorsal tarsometatarsal ligaments
Dorsal metatarsal ligaments
Dorsal cuneocuboid ligament
Cuboid bone
Dorsal calcaneocuboid ligament

Right foot: medial view

Deltoid ligament {
Posterior tibiotalar ligament
Tibiocalcaneal ligament
Tibionavicular ligament
Anterior tibiotalar ligament
}
Dorsal talonavicular ligament
Navicular bone
Dorsal cuneonavicular ligaments
Medial cuneiform bone
Dorsal intercuneiform ligament
Dorsal tarsometatarsal ligaments
1st metatarsal bone
Tuberosity
Tibialis anterior tendon
Tibialis posterior tendon

Tibia
Medial talocalcaneal ligament
Posterior process of talus
Posterior talocalcaneal ligament
Calcaneal (Achilles) tendon (cut)
Sustentaculum tali
Long plantar ligament
Plantar calcaneo-navicular (spring) ligament

Injuries easily take place because of the structure and built in mobility. Leg lengths also influence the weight bearing of the ankles. If there is a short limb, then the stride will be longer for that limb, thus putting the ankle at a mechanical disadvantage because there will be a lateral motion accompanying. This will result in continuing incidence of ankle sprains for the short side. No amount of bracing can make up for the mechanical disadvantage in this scenario. The main idea here is to check the leg lengths for inequality, especially in the growing population.

Ankle sprains can occur at the inside of the ankle and the outside of the ankle from sports and other traumas. The typical ankle sprain is an inversion injury which injures the ligaments on the outside of the ankle. These tend to heal spontaneously though they can be severe or recurrently symptomatic necessitating treatment. The treatment we have devised is conducted without bracing or casts. We use ice massage and ultrasound and steroid injection to the most severely injured area. The ice massage helps to control swelling while the ultrasound promotes flexibility of the ligament tissue. The steroid helps to control the inflammatory change that the injury caused and reduces pain. This approach decreases the treatment time dramatically and shortens the rehabilitation time. A weight bearing film is taken as soon as the ankle improves.

Flat foot is seen when the medial longitudinal arch collapses with weight bearing. This is the result of the calcaneus, or heel bone, moving laterally on the talus. We usually note a tightness of the lateral ankle ligament structures which causes the calcaneus to shift. The secondary effect is for the first toe to be forced into a lateral configuration, placing increased stress on the first metatarsal-phalangeal joint, or the base of the big toe. The result is the well known bunion. The surgery for this problem is very good, but bunions are caused by another factor which is not addressed by that procedure. We have developed an approach to treat this by mobilizing the lateral talo-calcaneal joint using an exercise program and a special insert that forces the talus to come to normal. Keeping the talus in normal position causes the foot to maintain its arch. The bunion tends to slowly revert itself, and the pain for which most people get operated can be relieved locally. Working with each painful joint in the area promotes the normal mobility which is required for normal weight bearing.

The foot is painful occasionally because of the intrinsic muscles of the toes cramping. These small muscles lie between the metatarsals in the foot and move the toes in a side-to-side fashion. A classic example of this injury is the woman who wears high heels and takes them off after work, and rubs her toes. The underlying injury is a small enthesitis, or inflammation of the muscle-bone connection. The treatment for this is to isolate the muscle by palpation and to inject it or use ultrasound on it with a stretching exercise. Pain between the toes is often diagnosed as a Morton's neuroma. It is thought that the small nerves get injured and as they regenerate they ball up into a painful neuronal mass. This is a rare occurrence. Much more common is the injury to the intrinsic muscles noted above. I recently examined a pro golfer with an eighteen year history or foot pain of this nature. She was seen by many specialists, but refused surgery. We were able to relieve her pain in one session of treatment.

Many patients have swelling of the lower leg, foot, and ankle. This can be caused by a number of problems, the most familiar of which is the calf vein clot. This has gained much notoriety lately as public awareness has increased. An ultrasound test quickly rules this from consideration if the veins are found to be patent. Failure of the kidney, liver and cardiac organ systems must be ruled out as well. We have found that a little recognized cause of calf swelling is an enthesitis of the calf muscle. This tight area of muscle bone connector causes the serum portion of the blood to be blocked from going through the muscle causing the edema. Chronic edematous calf tissue loses the soft pliability of normal skin. The proteins in the edema fluid cause a toughening and thickening and discoloration of the affected areas known as brawny edema. As this process continues the skin continues to change toward a deep dermal fibrosis. The treatment is to mobilize the enthesitic area by a stretching exercise in conjunction with local steroid injection to the most painful areas. Immediate improvement is seen, that is in a day or two. In this example case below, a truck driver with longstanding knee pain and calf swelling came to see me for his knees. As you can see, the foot is warm and the color is normal, thus eliminating the artery and vein from consideration. On follow up after the injection procedure, wrinkles are appreciated in the anterior calf with dorsiflexion, indicating that there is now redundant skin from mobilization of fluid. It is possible that the dermal fibrosis and discoloration is a result of hydrostatic pressure in the calf where the skin is closest to the tibia, that is, anteriorly and inferiorly.

Another common diagnosis for those with foot pain is plantar fasciitis. This fascia extends from the heel bone to the base of the toes. The plantar fascia is thought to get stretched when the longitudinal arch flattens with weight bearing causing pain. For many years people were treated for spur formation at the front part of the heel where the plantar fascia inserts into the bone. Several years ago it was determined that these spurs are not reflective of heel pain nor do they mean heel pain is imminent. It is thought that the calcium forms in the fascia at the site of inflammation at the fascia bone connection site. Practitioners will continue to treat the anterior heel for pain however. The results of treatment are not very good and consist of repetitive local injections, casting, bracing, and surgery. Surgery was found to be particularly ineffective and plantar fascia release is no longer commonly performed. The reason that the treatments are not effective is that the source of the heel pain is not the fascia, but up in the ankle at the talo-calcaneal ligament. A trauma or misuse of the ankle causes an enthesitis of the ligament which manifests as pain while weight bearing. This ligament formation can be several inches long. The point to make here is that this ligament can be treated with deep heat or local steroid injection to limit the inflammatory response and improve flexibility. Commonly, morning pain is present. The pain will decrease as the ankle is used, but tends to return after a period of idleness such as sitting. We have treated many feet and ankles after failures of treatment elsewhere. A physiological evaluation of this last weight bearing organ of the body will help a great deal before surgery is attempted.

Chapter 11
Elbow and wrist pain

The elbow joint is more than just a simple hinge. This joint is mainly made by the connection of the ulna bone, one of the forearm bones, to the humerus, or arm bone. It is secured by connective tissue that is constructed to allow 180 degrees of extension to allow you to open your arm to straight. This connective tissue allows you to normally flex your elbow to 135 degrees for carrying objects. The other joint involved is the articulation between the radius, which is the other forearm bone, and the humerus. This joint allows you to rotate your wrist from palm up to palm down. The radius moves around the ulna during this motion. This joint is also secured by connective tissue. Remember, connective tissue, when healthy, allows normal motion and also limits motion at the extremes of the normal range of motion.

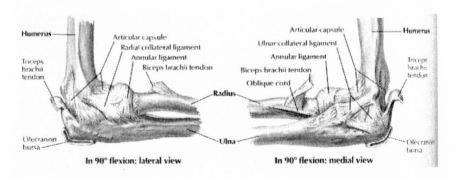

In 90° flexion: lateral view   **In 90° flexion: medial view**

These joints are controlled by surrounding muscles. Some of the muscles that control the wrist and fingers are located here. If you put your palm toward the ceiling the muscular bulge on the outside of the elbow will be the extensors of the wrist and fingers, the muscles that straighten the fingers and bend the wrist backward as if stopping traffic. The muscular bulge on the inside of the elbow will be the flexors, the muscles that curl the fingers and wrist. Common injuries to these muscle groups are an enthesitis-type injury, the pull injury on the muscle fiber insertion into the bone. If the flexors are involved it is called a "golfer's elbow", and if the extensors are involved it is called a "tennis elbow". I don't think either injury has anything to do with the sport they are named after. One important fact to never forget—maximum grip strength requires the wrist to be slightly extended. Watch what you do when you pick up a glass or a can of soda. You will see that your wrist extends as a part of the normal motion-pattern for grip! You need your extensor muscles to be functioning without pain for a normal grip. If you cannot extend the wrist due to muscle pain at the elbow, grip strength will be decreased.

The history that I take entails questions related to these functions outlined above. Can you open a jar, or carry a gallon of milk? Is there tingling in to the wrist or fingers? If so which fingers? The little finger tingling can be from the ulnar flexor muscles, and tingling towards the thumb is from the radial flexor muscles. Carpal tunnel syndrome, affecting nerves, has a different history, and the nerves can be checked easily enough by nerve conduction studies.

On examination, it is important to distinguish capsular pain form muscular pain. This is accomplished by documenting the extension of the elbow by measurement. If the extension is limited due to pain, then the capsule is affected. If not, then only the muscle cover is affected. Both can be painful in one elbow. If there is a muscle pain, known as an epicondylitis for where the muscle inserts into the bone, palpation of the muscular bulges will reveal if there is pain. Sometimes a patient will not think the elbow is the culprit but the history will suggest this finding and the examination confirms it.

In the past, elbow treatment entailed surgery. Now, I follow a new protocol with astounding success. The treatment undertaken depends on which structure is primarily painful. Usually the capsule is the most important structure to return to normal motion. This is accomplished by deep heat and minimobilization over several days, or local steroid injection will certainly and predictably return the motion to normal as the inflammatory condition is treated usually over one to two days. Muscular enthesitis injuries are treated through injection and ultrasound. We recommend an exercise program. As a basic tenet to follow, a muscle injury should be mobilized while a capsular/ligament injuries are to be stretched. I have had several excellent golfers and tennis players attain normal games after this approach. We are talking about days, not weeks or months of treatment.

An important caveat about elbow epicondyle injection for muscle pull injuries is that location is everything. It takes several minutes sometimes to isolate the most tender spot along the side of the elbow. Once this spot is found it needs to be confirmed by palpating the surrounding areas again. When injecting this area the physician *must* hit the bone with the needle. If the needle does not strike the bone, the symptoms may abate but there will be no cure. I have seen many individuals who were treated with elbow injections prior to coming to see me but without lasting cure. It is my belief that the precise area was missed and the pain did not resolve. Physicians will debate whether local steroid injections are beneficial for elbow complaints, especially epicondylitis, for this reason.

Carpal tunnel syndrome is the most common nerve entrapment syndrome in the body. The symptoms are numbness and tingling in the fingers of the hand, usually the thumb and first few digits. If severe enough there will we weakness in the thumb as well. The palm should not be affected though people may state that their whole hand is numb. Usually the symptoms will be worse at night and in the early morning as people will tend to sleep with their wrist bent, an exacerbating position for this condition. Those with CTS may show decreased sensory acuity in the thumb and index and long fingers when examined. Again, weakness will be noted in the thumb if severe enough.

The median nerve is located in a bony canal with 10 separate tendons around it, seen in the picture below. The roof of this canal is the volar carpal ligament. If there is too little room in the canal and the pressure on the nerve is too great, then the nerve begins to malfunction. The health of the median nerve is assessed by nerve conduction studies, as previously stated. If the nerve conducts too slowly, then the diagnosis of CTS is made.

Commonly people with this syndrome are treated with wrist braces and NSAIDs, and possibly referred for surgery if these simple treatments do not work. The surgical approach is to cut the carpal ligament to lessen the pressure on the nerve. We do not like the use of braces or splints for treating carpal tunnel syndrome because they hinder motion and the surgery causes a large scar. Our approach is to soften the carpal ligament by injecting a steroid to the areas of the carpal ligament where it attaches to the bone. This allows the ligament to increase its flexibility, thus decreasing the pressure in the carpal tunnel. The nerve then heals and allows normal conduction. We like this method as there is no scar, no time off work, no activity restriction, and no post-surgical pain. We have tested the median nerve before and after this kind of treatment and have shown a return of nerve conduction speeds along with diminished symptoms with this approach.

I must mention the long running commercials for arthritis of the hands by a drug company. The hands shown on that commercial are normal. The aching that took place for that person was actually elbow muscle pain. The treatment of that is to mobilize the muscle tissue that you will find to be painful on examination.

Chapter 12
Sports injuries

There are several aspects of sports medicine with which the reader should be familiar. The training aspect should be separated from the injury, in that the ideal candidate for training should be correct musculoskeletal-wise. There should be no restriction of motion of any joints, including spine motion, and no scoliosis or short limb. Each athlete must adhere to the principles of weight bearing described earlier. There should be no restriction on training, except that each and every sport has its own requirement for excellence.

If you are conducting a stretching program before sports, you should know that muscles normally stretch. The actual tissue that you are stretching is ligamentous. This activity raises body temperature, which improves the stretchability of the ligament on a temporary basis. Overstretching of the ligament at that time will also provide a temporary improvement. I feel that raising the body temperature before sports is the ideal program, which can be done by push-ups, sit-ups, and squats. Try it, it works.

When a restriction or reduced range of motion of any part of the body occurs, then an adequate physical exam will show this, and then correction of the problem could occur. This could only be done by qualified physicians who know how to examine properly and are knowledgeable in physiology. All age children and adults have the same injuries and conditions. Age has no special meaning when dealing with this concept of injuries.

One should not be impressed with the million-dollar athletes having the surgery du jour, and then relating it to your own family. There are many games played on and off the field by the teams and athletes. The usual arrangement of the medical staff on these teams is that there is a trainer and helpers and the orthopedic surgeon. Musculoskeletal physicians are nowhere to be found. It should be remembered that surgeons spend every day in their training period learning how to operate. Operative skills need to be developed and honed in those few years, for it is a great responsibility they hold in their hands. However, surgeons do not learn how to treat these problems non-operatively during those years. I routinely see orthopedic surgeons referring their patients to the physical therapist, who treat these people for weeks without physician supervision and focus on muscular imbalance instead of mobility. The health care arrangements for athletes are actually pretty poor in my opinion, with the only sure loser to be the injured player. Rarely do I hear of the exact diagnosis of the injury in these athletes. Usually, it is made by MRI and not by close examination. The elements described elsewhere in this book, of the knee for example, are rarely mentioned. It is always gigantic in importance.

A hands-on physician, not the surgeon, would be instrumental in saving these million dollar players from excessive surgery and disability. It is a rare athlete who is returned to pre-injury performance after surgery. Even if they return for a short time, their longevity is precluded. This is bad management on the part of the team owners.

The ideal treatment of most sports injuries is to quickly limit the inflammatory response of the tissue injured, which is usually ligament or enthesis. We do this by a close, detailed examination of the injured part, followed with an injection to this area with a non-residue steroid. The object is to decrease the response of the body to produce swelling and pain in the area. The swelling and pain is a natural result of injury and inflammation. Left untreated the natural repair process will produce scar formation and calcification of the injured part. If we can eliminate inflammation early and fully, then the natural response of the body is abrogated. You have then a soft pliable ligament and joint structure that will heal faster, without a scar. Ice and heat are not sophisticated approaches any longer. My athletes recover in a few days.

Each sport has its own body requirements and each should be trained and examined for that particular sport. Football players need different approaches than a baseball pitcher. Long distance runners have different needs than a sprinter.

Sports injuries in children and young adults are the same as for older people with some special needs of the growing child. The evaluation and treatment of these injuries, short of fractures, is essentially the same. We may not use steroids as much, but in the very young they are not needed because the tissues are more treatable. All children involved with sports should be examined in the same musculoskeletal way, especially for scoliosis and tight hips, low back and neck, and shoulders.

We have developed an accurate program for golfers. This entailed going back to the construction of the swing, and studying the tissues necessary to accomplish the swing and to keep it fluid and forceful. We have been using the program for a few years now and had the opportunity to treat a few professionals with pain. They were impressed. This program is good to go now. Essentially I view the golf game as a medical problem and as a skills problem. In other words, the medical aspect allows you to be a good golfer, and the skills for golf are taught by the professional. If you have limited torso rotation from an injury, then the professional will not be able to help your game. Both aspects need each other for maximum benefit to the game.

> "...my back has never felt better. I never realized how much pain I was actually in until I received my [treatment]. As a professional golfer, my back takes a beating from all the practice of beating balls and traveling. After seeing you I played in the Colorado Open. The weather was absolutely miserable—cold, rainy, windy, and tornado warnings everyday. Usually my back would feel tight in a situation like this but I felt loose and had more range of motion in my golf swing than ever before. I had my best tournament finish in over 2 years—19th place. The tournament brought massage therapists in for us and I am always the first in line. This time, I really didn't feel a need to go over there but it was free and I had the time. The

therapist said I did not have any knots in my back unlike all the other players who complained of tightness. I can't thank you enough for all your help and am hoping you come to Boca [Raton]—it's where you belong!"

D.S.—Boca Raton, FL

Recently I took care of a marathon runner who was having lateral knee pain toward the end of his race. This most likely would have been diagnosed at Iliotibial Band Syndrome or a knee sprain by another physician. What he actually had on examination was a medial hip capsulitis on that side, which caused the entire lower limb to assume an internally rotated position, which put more stress on the lateral knee and ITB insertion. We treated the hip and then the knee and his results were excellent. His testimonial follows:

"I started training for the Boston Marathon in November with a 50 mile first week and then increasing by 4 miles a week until I reached 86 miles. My workouts were going find and I saw my times on the 10 mile runs starting to drop from 1:07 to around 1:00 flat. The weather was a key factor as we had a brutal winter but I kept plugging along knowing it would all be worth it come April.

At the end of February I was on my typical 15 mile run on Saturday when I hit mile 11 and felt a pain on the outside of my knee. Thinking I aggravated something I plugged along and finished with my normal time on that run. Then Monday came along and I felt the same pain at around mile 9 this time...again I just continued along. Finally about three weeks later, with the pain not easing and starting to hit my knee earlier and earlier along in the runs I went to see Dr. Pannozzo. I told him I have 20 days until Boston, and I put my time and training in him and told him about my discomfort in the knee area. With his knowledge of Sports Medicine he then started to diagnose my situation.

We started out by taking some X-Rays and examining them. He then pointed out to me that my one knee was about ¼ inch higher than the other and said that after so much repetition on that leg eventually something would have to give. I could see that my hips were also a little

115

offset, not ¼ inch but a little bit. He told me that in order to reduce the pain in my knee I needed to start at the point that was initiating the pain and not just the source. With this we came up with some stretches and lifting for my upper leg/hip to help fix what was wrong up there first and that would fix my knee at the same time. I had 20 days to go so I started out with my stretches and lifting daily. I also received a few natural shots that would help out in the healing process. I continued to run and did my last race before Boston down in Columbus. I ran an awesome time which was where I needed to be for Boston and most importantly felt no pain in my knee. I was very nervous going into this race about my knee hurting, but it held up just fine and the treatment I received seemed to be working so Boston was looking brighter.

With 1.5 weeks to go before Boston, I picked up the miles for the last week and then slowed down my training a few days before the big run. I stuck with my stretches and lifting just like the doctor told me to and I got one more shot a few days before the big day. As I was at the starting line and had adrenaline going though my system I did think about my knee and hoped that nothing would go wrong and as I crossed the finish line with no pain in my knee I realized the treatment I have received and the stretches and lifting worked to perfection. I feel that if I did not go see Dr. Pannozzo and start the treatment from the hip and not the knee that I may have not finished in the top 1% at Boston. His wisdom of Sports Medicine and assessing the problem at where the beginning point is and not the source really helped me along in my healing. So with the right type of treatment and a few days to allow the results to kick in, I think any pain can be healed in time for anyone's big race!"

S.F.—Youngstown, Ohio

Another case recent case is of a 12 year-old baseball pitcher who was struck in the front of the knee by a ball. He limped from pain for 2 weeks. The examination of the knee showed that the knee itself was normal in every way except for the patellar tendon as it inserted into the tibia on the medial side. In addition, there was a hip flexion contracture present preventing the knee from fully extending as it was designed to bear weight, causing excessive pull on the patellar tendon. We first treated the hip flexion contraction and then the patellar tendonitis. This took 2 days to accomplish, with total function of the knee and hip without pain.

Sports injuries are easily treated if the basic concepts we have mentioned in previous chapters are adhered to during diagnosis and treatment. "Sports Medicine" is actually a marketing concept. Injuries are the same, no matter if you are diving for a line drive or falling down the steps. The body has the same components, same anatomy, if you are a running back or a salesman. Diagnosis and treatments are also the same. I am disappointed and dismayed when I read about athletes being rehabbed for a year for a groin injury, or an athlete traded to another team because of an injury that is easily treated, if you know how.

Warming up exercises have been studied extensively. The consensus now is that they are not productive. Why? Because the muscles are not stretched in the stretching exercises, but the ligament structures are stretched. Ligaments function better when warm, so if the temperature of the body is increased by exercises such as squats and push-ups and sit-ups, then the stiffness disappears. Over stretching of the ligaments causes injuries and pain noted the next day. If the stiffness persists, then a medical exam needs to be done to treat the cause of the persistent stiffness.

Chapter 13
The Ideal Pain Clinic

The ideal pain clinic for the consumer, which I am also, is the one that is oriented to cause and effect relationships for musculoskeletal pain syndromes. The idea is to prove each and every diagnosis. Unfortunately this idea usually gets corrupted between the concept and the end product. Today pain management clinics focus on a multi-disciplinary model, so that physical therapists, chiropractors, psychologists, surgeons and others add their knowledge to the treatment protocol. While this sounds quite good, it becomes apparent that if one from the group knew how to approach the problem correctly, the others would be unnecessary. Too often patients get stuck in a holding pattern, on a pain pill with a generic exercise program, waiting to see what comes next. Transferring your care to a therapist, manipulator, or psychologist is detrimental to solving your pain. A failure means a referral to the surgeon, an increase of the medications, or worse. This will sound all too familiar to those who have been there.

What we can make clear is that the problem occurs early in the usual path. The patient will be evaluated initially by a physician, maybe an anesthesiologist or a physiatrist. Unfortunately that patient will usually get saddled with a general diagnosis like cervical sprain or myofascial pain. This is the early problem that does not allow proper and effective treatment. It needs to be made crystal clear that if there is no specific diagnosis there can be no specific treatment. General treatments like an exercise program, manipulation, or the like will never offer efficient treatment like we are all looking for. The cause of the pain is the primary area to treat, but you must have a diagnosis. You must have a target for your treatment. This principle is widely accepted by physicians, yet they routinely accept "lumbar sprain" as an acceptable diagnosis.

The ideal pain clinic can reduce your pain in one to two days, if they know what they are doing. Most pain clinics will emphasize "realistic goals" and have psychological evaluation to find depression and convince the patient that he or she should accept the pain. This is not necessary and in my opinion this should be condemned. The clinics that emphasize psychology and psychological drug therapy are sadly missing the point, which is that effective treatment improves sleep disturbance, mood disorders, and the like.

There is also more to a pain clinic than easy prescription of drugs such as narcotics or muscle relaxants, or being a procedure mill, where the patient can get the "best" new treatments. Some clinics will offer the gamut of procedures, from epidurals to the newest, IDET. In the most recent study, IDET outcomes at 1 year after procedure are a failure. Newer is not always better. Epidurals should only be performed if there is true radiculopathy by EMG testing, though we unfortunately have seen these performed on those without. The point is that procedures do not help if the diagnosis is incorrect. If you are offered drugs, asked to change jobs, or you are asked to go for physical therapy or be off work for long periods of time, you are obviously in the wrong place. Giving you a disability is not the answer to a better life. The skills of the physician are the critical area to concern you.

The ideal pain clinic should be able to prove outcomes on a scientific basis. This is the ultimate proof that validates the treatment method and the physician's skills at diagnosis and treatment. The current standard is to accept the patients estimate on a line chart, called the Visual Analog Scale. Other times the patient is asked how they are able to do certain activities and a "number" is estimated from how well the patient states they perform, which is supposed to be a method of measuring outcome. Still another method is for the patient to look at a range of smiley faces, from sad to happy, and pick out which facial expression most fits their current emotional state.

119

As you may have guessed we find no science in these methods. The examination needs to document change in range of motion, which will be the ultimate guide to show improvement or not. If the person can bend only 70 degrees before treatment and then 90 degrees after treatment, than that is the way to prove improvement. If the patient can bend 90 degrees with pain prior to treatment, he should be able to bend full without pain after treatment. The point we are trying to impress is the initial exam must reproduce the pain, and then all future examinations must compare the current findings with the past. This is how a scientific judgment is made. This is entirely reasonable yet not done in most places.

The ideal pain clinic as we have produced will treat the cause of pain in days, not weeks or months. The basis is the range of motion exam and the specific history germane to your pain problem. Specific exercises based on that structure will decrease the pain. Each and every structure in our body has a pain pattern associated with it. I have spent my professional life unraveling these pain patterns. Our outcome studies are there for anyone to see.

The ideal pain clinic will not use IDET, manipulation, narcotics, or acupuncture. The ideal clinic will not espouse epidurals, surgery, or radio-frequency ablations, which is the burning of nerves. It will not call for procedures to implant wires or stimulators in your spine, or to implant a morphine pump, or other self medication gizmos, or promote meditation, yoga, physical therapy or water therapy, hypnotism, stabilization exercises or any other non specific treatment that was just listed. You want what I want, that is to be treated on a scientific basis, that is, to be able to predict improvement. Short of this, you will not improve.

The idea here is that there are only five structures that can cause pain. Many times there is an interaction among these five structures. The physician trained in musculo-skeletal physiology can distinguish the elements causing pain to be treated. The ideal pain clinic will have essential diagnostic and treatment facilities. The premises will operate as a physician's office having a business office for identification of patients and records. Several examination rooms should be present for taking of histories of the pain problem and then to do a physical examination. An in house x-ray is extremely important to save time for the patient and to get immediate results from the film to reduce the pain.

In addition electromyography and nerve conduction studies must be done as a service of the pain clinic. The physicians must be trained for this testing. Laboratory testing of blood can be done out of the clinic. An in house CAT or MRI is desirable but not necessary. Informational packets and exercise programs must be taught to the patients in detail. Specific treatments are to be done as part of the workup of the pain problem. These procedures are physician services. No physical therapy or other services are necessary. An in house training program must be given for technicians to help the physicians with their procedures and treatments. The pain clinic must take the patient seriously, and to produce a decrease in pain as fast as possible. Anesthesiologist services and orthopedic and rheumatologist services are not necessary in a pain clinic. Physical Medicine and Rehabilitation trained physicians are the core of the medical staff.

The history and clinical examination must be of the commitment type. To explain further, one cannot diagnose and treat a symptom or set of symptoms that are not clear and precise. The patient must be guided into a description of not only where the pain is located, but when it occurs. No pain is present always. Pain is always lateralized to one side or the other to be more severe. To have a clear history is to have the commitment of the patient. To elicit an adequate and precise history of the pain, there must be awareness on the part of the physician of the anatomy and physics of motion using the structures that could cause pain. A vast knowledge of not only bone structure and joints, but muscle origins and insertions and the nerve system that serves them is necessary.

Likewise, the physician cannot treat a source of pain that is not clear and precise on the clinical examination. The physician must commit himself to treat a specific source of pain or sources of pain to the patient. This is the only honest way to serve the patient. If more than one source of pain is identified, then the worst pain is treated that day, and lesser pain is treated in subsequent sessions. This program is outlined to the patient, so that there is complete cooperation with the program. Drugs, besides the anti-inflammatory type cannot be used in this clinic as they would be counter productive. As the treatment progress, normal activity for the patient is encouraged. One cannot identify structures for treatment that do not show that they are symptomatic.

In the last analysis of the pain clinic, persistence is the key to good results because there are so many parts involved.

Outcome studies are extremely important when discussing results of the approach to pain of the ideal pain clinic. It should not use the visual analog scales, but use specific questionnaires related to the pain problem that was treated. This is currently not done. The normal range of motion without pain is the ultimate goal of all diagnosis and treatment. Without the normal range of motion without pain, of the body part treated, the experience of the patient is a failure. There should be more credibility of the clinic and physicians. The so called multidisciplinary clinic is in reality a machine without a motor. No head means no coherent thrust of the treatment for the patient.

Chapter 14
Temporomandibular Joint Pain

TMJ, the common name for pain from the temporomandibular joint, is a real source of pain. I have seen many patients with complaints of face pain. Some of these patients have real joint pain and some had pain radiating form the base of the skull. This joint may be located just in front of the ear on the side of the face. This joint is the link between the lower jaw and the skull. It is the "hinge" which allows us to open our mouths widely to eat a hotdog or to let a dentist peer at our teeth. There is a temporomandibular joint on each side of our heads.

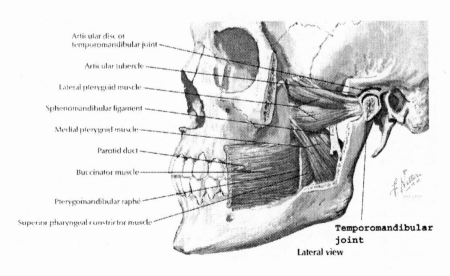

Articular disc of temporomandibular joint
Articular tubercle
Lateral pterygoid muscle
Sphenomandibular ligament
Medial pterygoid muscle
Parotid duct
Buccinator muscle
Pterygomandibular raphé
Superior pharyngeal constrictor muscle

Temporomandibular joint
Lateral view

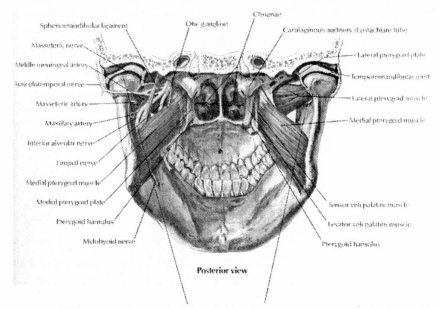

Choanae

Sphenomandibular ligament — Otic ganglion — Cartilaginous auditory (Eustachian) tube

Masseteric nerve

Middle meningeal artery

Auriculotemporal nerve

Masseteric artery

Maxillary artery

Inferior alveolar nerve

Lingual nerve

Medial pterygoid muscle

Medial pterygoid plate

Pterygoid hamulus

Mylohyoid nerve

Lateral pterygoid plate

Temporomandibular joint

Lateral pterygoid muscle

Medial pterygoid muscle

Tensor veli palatini muscle

Levator veli palatini muscle

Pterygoid hamulus

Posterior view

Illustration showing the two temporomandibular joints.

The history is extremely important here. When discussing the normal physiology of this joint, one must be aware of the function of this joint, and to realize that there are two of them working in tandem to allow the excursion of the mandible to open the mouth for feeding and for speech. The joint itself is constructed as a knee, that is, with a joint capsule and cartilage. I have developed an accurate history for disorders of this joint based on the normal function of this joint. Any joint will have the symptom of stiffness in the morning, or after sleep. There are 3 questions in the history that are based on function. First question, then, is—Are you experiencing morning stiffness so that you have a pain when opening your jaw? Second question—Are you having trouble eating a hot dog? Third question—Is chewing on either side of your jaw painful? If the answer to each is yes, then TMJ is present. If the answers are no, then the pain is referred from another source.

It has been said that there may be spasm of the muscles surrounding the joint. This is not critical thinking, because the muscle pain should be regarded as guarding, the resistance of motion to prevent pain. The examination entails evaluating both sides at once. We test the excursion of each joint to elicit not only the pain, to reproduce it, but to test the excursion of the joint and to palpate the restriction of motion and the looseness of motion for each side. This technique leads the physician to treat the restricted side. This is in keeping with the general principles of musculoskeletal evaluation. This method will restore the normal range of motion without pain. There is however an underlying cause of the syndrome, and that is the bite. Here we work closely with a dentist who is skilled in evaluating the bite and to correct it. I have seen patients with a scar around this joint from a previous surgery. This makes the treatment more difficult but the principles are the same—mobilize the restricted side.

This treatment can be accomplished by applying ultrasound to the joint with a minimobilization, or local injection with a steroid followed by the ultrasound and minimobilization. The results are uniformly good. There is no place in the regime for treatment for biofeedback, drugs of any kind or psychological treatment. Stress of any kind will not produce pain in this small joint. We should not ever impugn the patient as having "stress" as this is an untenable idea. People do not have stress causing a local phenomenon, but the stress occurs between the ears, that is, mental and it stays mental. Another possible source of jaw pain is the insertion of the flexor of the jaw as it attaches to the maxilla, and is an inflammation of the muscle bone connector. This area is also treated locally with good results. We should not forget that some patients will have a referred pain from cardiac reasons. Other sources of face pain are located at the C_0-C_1 and C_{1-2} vertebrae. There is no science in posture training or strengthening muscles when they are not weak but only painful. Splinting the jaw with an expensive splint is to add into the problem of scaring of the painful joint. We adhere to the principle of mobilization in rehabilitation and not restriction. Forget distracting your nervous system or changing your diet. Get the thing treated, and get going with your life.

Case History

A 54 year-old woman presented for evaluation for left face pain, worsened with opening the jaw for eating and wearing her denture appliance. Her symptoms began in 1975 and worsened to the point she sought a surgical procedure, which left a scar on the left mandible, or lower jaw. On examination there was tenderness over the scar with abnormal motion of the TMJ joint, with limited motion of the right TMJ joint and a hypermobility of the left TMJ joint. The scar was mobilized using injection and mini-mobilization techniques and her pain lessened. We began treating the TMJ pain by approaching this as an overuse pain on the left from a restriction on the right.

The right TMJ joint was treated with ultrasound, mini-mobilization, and occasional local steroid injection to promote mobility and flexibility. She now wears her denture, her eating habits have normalized and treatments have become intermittent, usually 2-3 months apart. She is under good maintenance at this point.

One cannot overlook a tooth infection as part of the pain in the face or jaw. Pipe smokers may have some of the symptoms of this disorder. The treatment is the same.

Chapter 15
Myofascial Pain Syndrome and Fibromyalgia

Ever since President Kennedy was treated for back pain, there has arisen a whole industry surrounding what is described as myofascial pain and also what is now called fibromyalgia. Both these diagnoses have become much more common, and I believe indiscriminately applied to patients complaining of multiple pains. There are physical therapy centers that are filled with patients diagnosed with a myofascial syndrome, and I have noticed a large number of publications devoted to fibromyalgia. It seems that the people with these diagnoses are looking for answers and treatment, yet they are not given them. I have reviewed the available material for these conditions prior to writing this book, and remain unimpressed with the author's science and understanding of these syndromes. I have seen thousands of people that were diagnosed with Myofascial Pain Syndrome prior to my examination then given a specific diagnosis afterward. I have seen thousands of patients who were diagnosed with Fibromyalgia prior to my examination then actually offered specific, treatable diagnoses. I hope people with these diagnoses read this chapter closely so that they can gain a new perspective on their ailments.

Physicians work in science as well as compassion. We must look for a cause and effect relationship for all complaints while offering our assistance. This cause and effect relationship is found in every part of the body. The effect of a disease or problem is reflected in the structure it affects—a bladder infection will show an inflammatory change in the bladder wall for example. Every disease you can think of, from cancer, to fungal infection, to herpes, to cirrhosis, <u>to a scar</u> has specific changes that are readily found under the microscope. In medical practice, there is always some way to verify pathology, via lab work or in the pathology lab. This must be accepted as fact or else there is no science in our efforts. There are only two diagnoses that I know of that do not have specific tissue changes under the microscope—Myofascial Pain Syndrome and Fibromyalgia. I will explain each diagnosis and point out what I have found to be different than what is accepted by the "experts", who may be less skeptical than me.

Myofascial pain and Myofascial theory has gained increasing prominence since the 1940s. Doctors were looking at painful areas in muscle since the 1800s, and this was gradually condensed into the Myofascial Pain Syndrome written about by Dr. Travell in 1942. Almost 50 years ago investigators were looking at painful muscles during electromyographic examinations, and they found areas with an electrical abnormality, a series of positive waves and polyphasic potentials, which are specific finding in electrodiagnosis. This work was felt to reflect the nature of the disease and the syndrome of myofascial pain was given credence. Later the electrodiagnostic findings were found to be *normally* provoked from certain *normal* places in the muscle, which was essentially a rebuttal of a major part of the basic tenets of the syndrome. It is now accepted that there are no abnormal electrical findings in the muscle. Nevertheless work continued steadily and soon a major two-part book was produced by Drs. Travell and Simons, of which I own a copy.

This book mentions references the Trigger Point (TP), the hallmark of myofascial pain. These physicians state that there are two kinds of trigger points, active and latent, that is silent. The active TP causes pain, and the latent does not—it just causes weakness and causes a loss of motion. I notice that there is no mention of how this TP forms from normal muscle, nor how an active TP becomes a silent one. As discussed in previous chapters, muscles contract and shorten to produce movement. This contraction is easily assessed with the electrodiagnostic examination. The EMG is normal in these patients; therefore there can be no weakness and motion loss—the muscle fires normally. There can be no argument for pain-related weakness from a latent TP. As you can see the science in this theory is lacking.

Another point is that there has been multiple muscle biopsy studies performed over the years, dating back to 1951. The trigger point nodules were found to be normal or have non-specific changes. There was no consistent finding that you would expect from a sequence of events that defines a specific disease. Drs. Travell and Simon state that repetitive puncturing of the TP with a needle is an effective method for treatment amongst other methods. I counter that there is no better way to make specific changes in a muscle than to keep injuring it and scarring it with multiple needlings.

Their book references the examination for trigger points and taut bands in the muscle by feeling these bands with your fingers. The proponents of Myofascial Pain Syndrome state that these trigger points are easily found as "ropiness" in the muscle tissue. I confess that I cannot feel them in spite of my large patient load. I question the fact that there is no other objective finding for this diagnosis. The simple fact is that I have always been able to diagnose other causes of pain in these patients. The pain patterns that have been mentioned in other chapters are entirely accurate. I personally have had a neck pain which referred pain toward the shoulder, causing the classic symptom of a tender muscle with trigger point. I had a colleague inject my facet joint. The neck pain, referred pain, muscle pain, and trigger point pain resolved with that treatment. With the points I have made above, it does not seem reasonable to me that Myofascial Pain Syndrome can be considered a true diagnosis by physicians.

There are some articles in the medical literature that try to make the distinction between Fibromyalgia and Myofascial Pain Syndromes. The difference is thought to be trigger points. The treatment of trigger points by injection is said to sometimes increase the range of motion of the joints. *This is of course impossible since the joint range of motion is controlled by the ligament structure or capsule of joint.* This is more proof that there is no scientific rationale for these entities.

Fibromyalgia has been an enigma for centuries. Years ago patients were diagnosed with "rheumatism", and it was not until 1976 that the word Fibromyalgia was first used. The diagnosis burst to prominence through the 1980's with AMA recognition of the diagnosis in 1987 and diagnostic "criteria" being established by the American College of Rheumatology in 1990. Fibromyalgia (FM) is diagnosed if a person complains of diffuse pain for three months and has pain with palpation in eleven of eighteen specific places. There are *no* other specific findings for this entity. There is no lab test or radiograph that can be ordered to show any abnormality. Any tissue examined under the microscope will look normal.

Lately researchers have tried to point to abnormal central nervous system processes or neurotransmitter dysfunction as a cause. Low levels of serotonin, a chemical in the brain, has been associated with this diagnosis. There is something called Substance P, a molecule that is released when a nerve is trying to transmit a pain impulse. Substance P has been found at high levels in people with Fibromyalgia. The body's stress system, the organs and hormones that help us cope with stress, has been found to be underperforming. There have been studies pointing to far many more lab work abnormalities, though none of these are as widely accepted. With all of these findings Fibromyalgia is a biochemical abnormality right? Not so fast. No one, certainly not me, is denying that these people have pain. But persistent, multiple injuries could be expected to do the same thing to Substance P levels. Medications that raise serotonin levels are not curative of this problem. The stress system connotes an emotional, psychogenic basis for FM, as the person's negative stressors overcome their ability to function. These individuals will tell you that they are not crazy, they do not have mental issues, and they only want you to get rid of their discomfort. Patients with this diagnosis are poor sleepers, which does not help the problem. One thing I agree with and will do for people with persistent, multiple pain complaints is to offer a medication to help them get a good, restful sleep. There are a few sedating medications available to help in this regard.

Once you start examining these patients and finding the source for these referred pains, it then becomes easy to offer a treatment regimen. One example I will offer is the pain in the middle of the back and referring under the shoulder blade. The diagnostic pain areas are on the scapula itself, but I have found this to come from the C_7-T_1 annulus. I treat this structure and that pain leaves. Another area is the first rib insertion of the scalene, or neck "strap" muscles. This will refer directly backward to the area between and above the shoulder blade. There are other areas like this that take a special examination to be found, where a physician carefully studies the area affected from all angles.

In the literature there is described a post-traumatic fibromyalgia, with the onset of diffuse pain. We should really look at this diagnosis with a skeptical eye. Trauma causes tissue damage, and it is up to the physician to find it. These people will have no indicators of muscle damage, like the elevated muscle enzymes or myoglobin in the blood. How can a normal person, after an automobile collision, for example, develop this new "disease" replete with central nervous system abnormalities, nerve receptor hyper-irritability, and neurotransmitter dysfunction and extreme muscle pain, all with no detectable changes? I believe it is much easier to understand that pain is coming from the muscular insertion, the muscle belly itself is *normal,* as expected by the normal laboratory findings, and in fact this is a misdiagnosis. My mentor, Dr. John Guyton, a physiatrist in Columbus, Ohio stated that there was no such thing as post-traumatic fibromyalgia, only post-traumatic misdiagnoses. I could not agree more.

Many times I find that the physicians making these diagnoses are unskilled in musculoskeletal pain problems. I have personally seen people diagnosed with fibromyalgia by their primary care physician without the appropriate exam to show eleven of the specific eighteen tender points. These primary care physicians, always pressed for time, sometimes will make a diagnosis based on what they are told without the appropriate objective findings.

Why is it important to document pain sources? Because patients are treated based on the diagnosis. First, most patients are treated with antidepressants or even narcotics, both of which I feel are contraindicated in pain because they do not treat any specific structure, just mask perception of pain. I think that a patient's mood will improve considerably if you treat their pain complaint. The assumption is that this pain is from "muscle," but muscles are not treated, except for water therapy or some generalized physical therapy program which is doomed to failure, thereby verifying that this disease is untreatable. It is self-fulfilling. Most patients that call me for these problems want drugs only. They are bombarded with information that says to them basically, there *is no help for you*. This attitude is found in many periodicals available to the general public, and added to by their health professionals when their doctor tells them to accept their pain. The support groups are merely social gatherings and centers for bad information.

We approach this problem as any pain problem, using the 5 tissues as sources of pain generators and examining each in turn to produce a diagnosis, and then to treat the area. This is the same approach I use in sports medicine or work injuries. We cannot make the musculo-skeletal organs to fit a different set of diseases. We are what we were designed to be. These devastating syndromes must be thrown out as a treatable disease state. To my mind there is no attempt to understand this problem. Those that write about this syndrome do not go far enough to determine the source of pain. They are bogged down with fascia or connective tissue or chemicals as the source of pain. I have gone beyond this as a source of pain to the moveable parts of the spine and other joints. Those writing about this problem admit that there may be trauma in the history but they cannot narrow the moveable parts as the source of guarding against motion of parts that are painful to move. To make this point clear, the body will prevent movement of a joint that is painful. This protection is guarding and not spasm or fibromyalgia.

Your takeaway idea here is to discard this diagnosis and to seek meaningful medical treatment. Range of motion exercises will give more relief than trigger point injection or drugs. Get an adequate examination of the structures that are painful such as the neck, or dorsal area or shoulder areas. Dieting is no answer to this painful condition. There are no inflammation-producing foods. A cheeseburger at McDonald's is the same meat that you serve as steak at home, just ground up. Fast food is the same as we serve at home, just faster and more convenient-thus the term fast food.

Entire books have been written about these two topics. We are able to condense this chapter to a few pages simply because the Fibromyalgia Syndrome does not happen.

A 56 year-old female complained of neck pain, headache, thoracic pain, and lumbar pain and was diagnosed with Fibromyalgia by her family doctor. She was given pain pills, anxiety medications, and anti-depressants for her symptoms and sent to physical therapy. She was tested with X-Rays, MRIs, and CT Scans, but she was not given a more specific diagnosis. Her biggest complaint was neck and shoulder pain when she came to see me after suffering for 8 years. On my examination her pain was localized to the C5-6 level, which refers pain to the shoulder blade. The shoulders themselves had a normal examination. This level was treated with injection and ultrasound, and on her next visit her neck pain had resolved and we moved on to her lumbar spine. There are scores of examples like this, where people suffer because of improper diagnoses. The point of this example is that there is a source for pain, and this source must be localized and treated specifically. Fibromyalgia is not a diagnosis, it does not mean permanent pain, and it should be forgotten, in my opinion.

Another case of a patient who was diagnosed with fibromyalgia was prescribed drugs down the line to narcotics. She was sent to rehab for drug abuse on two occasions. You can see that the original medical problem is now drug abuse.

Chapter 16
Complex Regional Pain Syndrome

Reflex Sympathetic Dystrophy (RSD)

Complex Regional Pain Syndrome (CRPS) is a relatively new term for the older diagnoses of reflex sympathetic dystrophy and causalgia. In general these syndromes are diagnosed when there are clusters of symptoms like pain, swelling, and blood flow changes in the upper limb or the lower limb. The primary difference between the two diagnoses is that CRPS type I, previously known as RSD, does not involve explicit nerve injury. CRPS type II, previously known as causalgia, does involve nerve injury, for example if a knife or bullet were to sever a nerve. The symptoms between the two subsets are similar, though no one is clear about how or why they develop, or how they are mediated over time.

Causalgia came to the forefront after the U.S. Civil War when the army physician Mitchell described a pain syndrome in veterans who suffered bullet wounds that damaged peripheral nerves. In the early 1900s Leriche was studying this syndrome and Charcot joints and began to study the sympathetic nervous system as a possible cause. Others followed and this concept has predominated until recently when new information has questioned whether the sympathetic nervous system has a role at all.

The primary symptoms of the CRPS syndromes are pain, swelling, and changes in movement of the limb. Some individuals may complain of altered sensation so that non-painful stimuli are painful and minimal painful stimuli cause excruciating pain. However, when a careful sensory exam is done, there is no evidence of sensory loss to fine touch. Going back to the 5 components of pain producer structures, this leaves ligament to consider. There may be a loss of range of motion of a joint involved in this syndrome, but the main component still causing pain on movement, and swelling, and edema, is the ever present enthesitis. This localized muscle inflammation and pain will cause all of the changes distal to it that are described in the literature. The conclusions in the literature, though, are not accurate. The literature suggests, but does not prove any cause.

Initial treatment for suspected CRPS is oral prednisone, usually a taper dose from 100mg to off over 10 days, decreasing 10mg per day. The concept of an exaggerated inflammatory response as the basis for this syndrome should be remembered and it needs to be treated aggressively. Along with the oral medication route, the local cause should be isolated and treated locally with mobilization and local injection to hasten the cure.

The treatments that are prescribed elsewhere are of mobilization of the area with physical therapy without isolation of the enthesitic locale. They are partially correct.

Over the years, I have seen many syndromes of this type and have devised a treatment regime to deal with all of the pathological appearances of the limb. The main thrust is to rule out any nerve or ligament signs. Then to carefully examine the limb for a local painful muscle-bone location of the most severe pain. The mobilization of this area can be accomplished by ice massage for 7 minutes, followed by ultrasound for 8 minutes, followed by the minimobilization that was described previously. There is no indication of sympathetic nerve system involvement directly. So, blocking the plexus is not going to help. Instead, if the symptoms warrant it, the main painful spot must be isolated, and injected at the muscle-bone connection with a short acting steroid and pain killer. This is then followed by the rest of the regime. Good results are predictable. Several attempts must be made to do this routine, because more than one place may be involved. The idea here for the public, is that this complex is made worse by those not initiated in this process and investigation. Anesthesiologists must refrain from being too aggressive in their approach. Musculo-skeletal specialists will have most of the answers on this syndrome. Narcotics have no place in this inflammatory problem Psychology and counseling is not indicated. Physical therapists and chiropractors are not equipped to treat this problem. Many times the family doctor or neurologist will prescribe uncontrolled therapy. The results will be disastrous for the patient. This is a treatable syndrome and you should get the best care possible. I noticed that many people carry this diagnosis, and are receiving disability payment. When this happens, then the situation and problem will not go away or be treated properly.

Chapter 17
Pain in Children

I have a good practice of treating children with pain. The history and physical exam must change however. If the child is mature enough, then they can give you a history as an adult would. If they are younger, and shy, then the mother or dad will give the history to you. Remember, the musculoskeletal system is the same for all ages. The younger the patient is, the more the exam takes place by observation from a distance and not hands on. The same principles apply though, which is, range of motion loss from pain. Young patients are flexible, so that the painful area is readily noted because of the range of motion loss. The painful areas that I have treated range from the neck-headache, to shoulder pain to dorsal pain from a scoliosis, to lower back and hip and knee pain and foot pain. The location of pain is not the most important aspect of children with pain however. The treatment is the most important consideration.

In the present practice, the pediatrician, and orthopedic surgeon usually consult with each other. The actual treatment is done by a physical therapist. When the treatment is appropriately done, surgery is less indicated. Bracing for a number of problems is related to restriction of motion, which is against my principles of rehabilitation which as you know by now is based on mobilization of tissue. I feel that these helpless children must be treated by my personal touch for optimal results in my office.

Osgood-Schlatter disease is merely a patellar tendonitis, and can be readily treated as such. A tendon is strengthened after the inflammation is contained, which is a very successful regime without bracing or other therapies. The trick here is to evaluate the hip function which affects the knee. Sports injuries are treated similarly, in that an athlete who injures his same ankle often, has a weight bearing problem and should have that analyzed, before surgery or anything else is contemplated.

Young children can have back pain as any adult. This is brought about by roughhousing, or falling, auto accidents, abuse at home, jerking of limbs, or unimaginable accidents. Remember, any child can develop a pain like any adult.

The concept of hypermobility necessitating surgery to tighten up the laxness is faulty. One must examine the joint for tightness in another area, and when found, to mobilize it. The lax tissue will tighten normally. This is the nature of ligamentous tissue.

Examination of the neck is done with great skill, by using objects to suggest to the child to look to the right or left and to record the degree of motion for example. Similarly the child is examined for the complete range of motion for each painful area such as the shoulder, hip, or knee, etc.

An x-ray is completed for fracture if one is suspected, and then the appropriate treatment is begun. Bracing is usually not necessary. Pain reduction is very quickly achieved, and is noted by the mother in activity at home, and by formal repeat examination.

The current system, used in many children's hospitals, is that the pediatrician consults with the orthopedic surgeon for a pain or growth problem in the child. The surgeon then turns the child over to a physical therapist to treat and report back to the surgeon. There is a disconnect between the surgeon and the therapist, because the therapist will treat the patient as he knows how to, which may not be the state of the art, therefore a lesser standard of care is possible. In our children's hospital, a pediatrician not trained in musculoskeletal medicine depends heavily on the physical therapist. Not a good idea.

Chapter 18
Pain in Cancer Patients

Cancer continues to be one of medicine's most difficult challenges. Investigators and oncologists have made great strides in the last 10 years in developing new medications and treatment protocols to give cancer patients optimal outcomes. Cancer is the growth and spread of abnormal cells, which if becomes extensive can result in severe morbidity and mortality. Over 1.3 million Americans will be diagnosed with cancer in 2004 as estimated by the American Cancer Society, and over 500,000 will die from their disease. Cancer is the second leading cause of death in our society.

Lives are changed when a diagnosis of cancer is made. Patients will stabilize their spousal, family, financial, and social matters in preparation for what may lie ahead. A realistic attitude with components of hope, courage, and an inner peace seem helpful for this period. What should not be lost in the emotional and planning times are that cancer patients are otherwise just like non-cancer patients and can injure themselves during activity. We all have joints and joint capsules, muscles and muscle insertions, ligaments and ligament insertions, and bones and nerves. While the physician must consider more potential diagnoses in a cancer patient, painful conditions are related to the cancer itself or its treatment maybe 15% of the time only.

Oncologists are generally excellent clinicians and perform quite well in their cancer treatments. However oncologists are not well trained at diagnosing and treating musculoskeletal pain conditions. I remember quite clearly a patient with lung cancer who came to see me for a severe shoulder pain which she developed while undergoing chemotherapy treatment for her malignancy. She complained earlier to her oncologist, but he refused to admit the possibility that the shoulder pain was not related to her cancer. The oncologist increased her narcotic pain medications to the point where she found it difficult to even stay awake during her last few months. She left the hospital to see me in my office. I examined the shoulder and relieved the shoulder pain as we do with shoulders. She was extremely grateful for the relief that she had obtained. This is a perfect example that we try to stress, that no matter what your underlying condition may be, perhaps, your painful condition can be treated successfully. It takes a skilled, trained physician to do this kind of evaluation and treatment that is to be able to distinguish normal "pain producing structure" and cancer pain.

There are only two instances where pain may be produced by a cancer:

1. A cancer located in an enclosed area, which will cause a stretch phenomenon as the growth continues.
2. A cancer in the bone which weakens it to the point of fracture.

There is therefore hope for people with pain that may not be cancer in origin. The usual evaluation must take place. The bone scan is the best diagnostic test for spread of cancer to other structures that can produce pain. There after, the normal musculoskeletal examination takes place to locate the source of pain which is usually musculoskeletal in origin. Drug therapy or exercise program or local injection will go a long way to making the cancer patient more comfortable in their remaining days. If other areas of pain are present, then appropriate regimens can be done. Scarring of tissue from radiation can also be treated in the same way, which is to promote the mobilization of that tissue. I do not believe in neuropathic pain caused by cancer attacking the nerve, except by proving it by appropriate testing.

Chapter 19
Alternative Treatments

As consumers of the health network, as you and I are, it is imperative that we be able to separate marketing from science in the information that we are bombarded with daily. Often I am embarrassed by claims made by groups associated with large universities touting some treatment or another without any backup whatsoever. For example, I just recently read that water therapy was beneficial for osteoarthritis, but no figures were given and no pre-examination for the patients was analyzed with the examination after the treatment. Only an opinion of beneficial effects was given. As you know, I have showed on these pages that there must be some proof given, which must be based on good science of the normal physiology of the musculoskeletal system and the failure of that system. Another example is my reading of "neuropathic pain". The research was conducted on patients with this diagnosis and conclusions were given. But the definition of "neuropathic" pain was completely the patient's description of the pain and not on a nerve pain medical model. The subjectivity of the patient and the lack of objectivity and skill of the researchers render the research and conclusions irrevelevant. All of the conclusions in this book are proven in clinical practice and will pass the test of double blind study.

No one should be treated for a painful condition using any type of mind altering drugs or psychological or psychiatric treatment.

Pain has a source, and it must be found. If pain is not evident in a clinical exam, then it cannot exist. The principle here is that there must be a range of motion loss for a musculoskeletal pain to exist.

I usually tell patients that water therapy is too general to treat a specific pain of walking. It makes no sense to me that a patient limps into the pool, then stays there for 30 minutes in a so called non-weight-bearing pool, then limps out and around for the next whole day. These patients are trying to cheat the surgeon, but good results of treatment do this, not water. Water is for cleaning and drinking.

Mind-body dissociation using yoga, moxibustion, meditation, getting other interests, ignoring pain, group therapy, common interest groups, and support groups have no scientific validity, that is, what is causing pain and how it causes it and how we can treat the source. Classes of Yoga and other disciplines of the Far East cannot treat the pain source with these general type exercises. These groups are for socialization only. The problem is that the authorities recommend these people to these programs simply to dispose of complaining patients for the most part.

The use of electrical stimulative devices is in the alternative treatment realm. Most of the manipulators and therapists use these devices for treatment of pain without having a nerve involved. Just putting an electrical current through a painful area cannot cure anything. Most of pain is ligamentous in origin as we have discussed previously in this book. Acupuncture has no scientific base. I recall listening to a representation of the benefits of this type of treatment. The physicians presenting the cases had not properly diagnosed the sources of pain in the examples provided. I happened to know what the proper diagnosis was.

Acupuncture in my opinion is no more that pinching the skin, causing a sensory phenomenon. There is no way this can treat the source of pain. Usually the one doing the acupuncture is not trained in musculoskeletal medicine and is not able to make the proper diagnosis. This fact obviated the whole presentation, and it was not worth the time to sit there. I walked out.

Epidural injections are in this category also. The procedure to instill a pain killer into the spine is not diagnostic and does not guarantee relief of pain. Therefore this procedure should not be done. Again, the source of pain is not treated; therefore the results are not positive.

Manipulation of the spine is in the alternative sphere of treatments for pain. There are two reasons that this approach will not work. The first is that the chiropractic discipline does not allow for a complete and accurate diagnosis. They follow the allopathic and osteopathic models, and then add manipulation to it. In my vast experience, cracking of the back and neck is to be discouraged. There is no cause and effect studies available to justify this approach to painful conditions. Most of the chiropractors have taken advantage of the worker's compensation laws to promote time off and milk the system for the injured worker. Many times the worker thinks he is beating the system, but in reality he is being defeated by the system. This promotes excessive testing and consultations and treatments that everyone knows do not work to cure the patient but to "prove" disability. These hapless people are seen in my office after many months and years of disability, and many times multiple surgeries, seeking to justify their claim because the system decided that "enough is enough" and that the claim is not going to be paid anymore.

Magnets are sold for the express purpose of relieving back pain. They cannot do anything for us. The wave form of the magnet is not strong enough to affect us. Secondly the magnet does not know where the pain source is located. Inflammation is not affected by magnets or electrical stimulation.

Lumbar supports will not treat the back pain because the general principle of mobilization is denied with back supports. They will not work in any case because the object is to prevent motion of the spine, and to do this requires bone to bone fusion.

Chapter 20
Industrial or Occupational Medicine

I have examined and or treated thousands of work-related injuries over the years. These range from headache to foot pain. These injuries are no different than any other musculoskeletal injuries. Any attempt to distinguish this type of injury from a home injury or auto accident will fail if the examiner does not adhere to the guidelines I have already written. That is, he or she must determine which of the five structures is responsible for a pain. Unfortunately, there is a legal system around this, protecting the work-related incident from being viewed as any other injury or medical problem. In Ohio, where I practice, the first diagnosis given by any health care worker is the final diagnosis. If the diagnosis is only part of the problem, or inaccurate, then it is almost impossible to treat the patient the correct way. It now becomes a legal problem, with the Managed Care Organization (MCO) expert involved. Most of the time, this person has an axe to grind and may vote against you, and I have several examples of this. A 32 year-old man with children once wanted me to treat him for a low back and hip injury. The MCO decided that their expert, not having seen the patient, did not feel that what I wanted to do was not approved. I showed them that the diagnosis was exact for the lumbar complaint, such as the L_{4-5} facetal capsulitis on the right. The MCO then sent him to another consultant that does not have an outpatient practice such as mine, who wanted this man to have stabilization exercises with out knowing exactly what was wrong with him. The patient wanted me to treat him and the MCO sent him to some physical therapist for this terrible system of exercises that is not related to structure. This regime takes more time and is not prospective, so that the whole experience was worthless for this patient. Politics, not science, rules in the Ohio Bureau of Workers Compensation.

There is a set of rules, the Milliman and Robertson guidelines, which set standards of care for state-paid, work-related claims. As we all know, no one patient can fall within the rules set down by this committee to set normal treatment times. However, the MCO and the nurse will deny treatment based on this dubious text. The text is dubious because it is not based on a real patient, but only a composite. It is someone's idea of how long a person should be painful for an individual diagnosis. No real treating physician can adhere to these rules. The patient always suffers when this happens because the MCO controls the case and will deny payment for further treatment. No one is accountable at the MCO level for a wrongful decision on treatment.

I have had 500 employees at one time in the nursing home business. I owned one 150 bed nursing home and another 200 bed skilled nursing home. I was the medical director and made myself the employee examiner. I complied with the ADA, by fitting the employee to the job so that they would not hurt themselves. I used the ideas that you are reading about here to take a good history and examination. I picked out many unqualified people because they were painful and hired many that would not hurt themselves. They appreciated the fact that I could be concerned about their welfare. For three of the last years that I owned these facilities, no reportable injuries took place. I was given a huge refund by Ohio because the premiums came down. To do this, I had to work with any physician or chiropractor who attempted to maximize the claim. In other words I knew what should be done, and the other side knew this to be true.

I had a radio program for several years, which was a call-in show about pain. One day an OSHA employee called me on the radio to discuss injuries on the job. He was adamant about changing the jobs, causing a great deal of money to be spent by the employers. So, I asked him a hypothetical question: If 50 men

145

were doing the same job and one got hurt, would it be the job or the man? This OSHA man thought the job should be changed—I disagree. The man was inappropriately hired for that job! This man had a predisposing condition for him to get hurt. Ergonomists are on quicksand I feel, because they do not have the clinical skills and knowledge of anatomy and the physiology of weight bearing to be effective.

We did two retrospective studies on my patients five years apart, using consecutive work-injured cases. The main criteria were: return to work without retraining, being off work, or changing to an intermediate job site. The studies both showed that 91% of these patients went to the same job without time off, retraining, or intermediate jobs. The 9% were deemed to be frauds because the injuries were not of the type that would require time off or retraining. Some retired. These studies are true, and reproducible. The system outlined in this book works very well.

In the first example, where the MCO consultant opined that the treatment was not going to be approved, no investigation by him took place. One call would have been good for that patient. This is not good medicine. In the OSHA story, government needs to have better science to do its job. A balanced approach to industry is appropriate.

The protocol that we developed, to diagnose and treat work-related musculoskeletal injuries can be taught to others. At least there would be a baseline on which to make decisions, and thus to take the work injuries from the untrained, and move them to those more skilled in accurate diagnosis and treatment. The injured patient will be the winner in every case, and the employer.

We recently had a patient who injured his lumbar spine while in Canada. He was sent to a local service, supposedly a spine institute. There he was told he would never return to his job again, and given narcotics and told to enroll in physical therapy. He came to see me on the following Monday, extremely painful but the history and clinical exam was quite clear. Our special film was taken and the approach to his diagnosis was outlined for him. Options were given. He chose the injection method. The first day, two injections were given and on the Wednesday following, two days later, the last two injections were given. On the next day, Thursday, he returned to full time unrestricted work. The treatment was done to specific areas and fully documented. This is service of the future and available now.

In my experience from treating so many patients injured on the job, it is quite evident that the company failed to place that injured worker in the appropriate job for his physical makeup. By this I mean that the overall evaluation of the job requirements and the proper worker was not a consideration. This is just plain ignorance of the physiology of weight bearing as I have described it earlier in this book. Industry leaders must stop hiring their friends or relatives for the medical director position, and instead learn on their own some of the needs of that the position. The medical director should be cognizant of the spine and how it is injured to stop future claims against the company. No one benefits from injuries. Perhaps the job should be put up for bid? The doctor should at least know something about musculoskeletal injuries. The executives I have met at conferences just throw up their hands in disgust and confusion about the state injury programs. Many owners of business refer workers to their chiropractor friends and then bemoan the losses. For example, a restaurant owner was complaining of his employee injuries, and on inquiry, he said he refers his injured workers to his neighbor, a chiropractor. If the results are good, then, fine. But to jeopardize your employees because you like your neighbor is nonsense.

There is a routine that I use to evaluate employees. First, I need to know what job is the individual being hired for now. Then, I need to know what is required in the way of lifting, or sitting or pushing, or walking. Next, I examine the musculo-skeletal system for pain in the range of motion of each part. If the job for instance, requires someone to sit and type, then the range of motion of the wrist is to be examined. In my experience Carpal Tunnel Syndrome does not occur from typing. Look for symptoms from the radial carpal joint.

On the employee part, I was impressed with the fact that some prospective employees know that they are painful, and plan to file an injury complaint after securing the job. I have seen many of them when running my own company. Another example, of an employee not fitted to the job is a person with scoliosis or pelvic obliquity hired

147

to bend and lift and to carry. This type of employee will get hurt, predictably.

There is emerging another strategy in which the family physician will refer a patient with an injury claim to a certain chiropractor for treatment as long as the patient will get his drugs from him. This works the other way also. I have been asked by chiropractors to be involved in this fashion. The answer is always no. I have had at least three calls per week to write prescriptions for drugs and the answer is always "no". I require the patient to be detoxified during the treatment phase in my office. The authorities should be aware of this situation and do something to eliminate it.

There are patients on disability for months and years. When they are seen in my office, they are very protective about their status of being on disability. One cannot take them away from that notion that they should be protected so that the monthly check will come in. Family doctors will keep these people on the dole by not asking those who can cure the disability to see them. I have had many examples of this happen to me and my service. These practitioners will continue to send these patients to services that they know will not tip over the situation and keep these people on the disability roles. If the bureau of workers comp is serious, this situation can change rapidly. But sending the patients for an assessment of disability percentage is tantamount to getting rid of them unless that physician is also a treating doctor.

When you read this section, it is intended to explain that work injuries are in the political area, and you should get your injury treated as soon as possible, because politically and financially, there is not enough money to be spent on these programs. You the patient will be the loser eventually.

Chapter 21
Medications for Pain Relief

Medications play a major role in pain relief and have been used in one form or another for thousands of years if not longer. Today's medications are better and safer than ever before. Patients with pain of some type are generally treated with anti-inflammatories of some kind, but occasionally not. Narcotics are used extensively depending on the cause and how severe the pain is reported to be. Other physicians will use muscle relaxers and anti-depressants or anti-seizure medications in this population as well.

As you may know by now I feel that only certain medications should be used for pain. Inflammation is the underlying process with all injuries and therefore anti-inflammatories should be used in all cases. Steroids are derivatives of the natural hormone cortisone. Cortisone has weaker anti-inflammatory ability and other side effects. This profile has been improved in the laboratory over the years leading to the various steroids available today. Prednisone, Medrol, and others are taken by mouth, usually in a tapering dose over a week. These are powerful agents and should be taken only under the supervision of a physician.

Injectable steroids have variable potency and two major preparations, which are short acting and long acting. I prefer a potent, short acting agent to any other variation. The drug is placed, has its softening effect, and then is cleared by the body. The drug's effect remains after the drug is cleared, make no mistake, but the drug does not remain to continue to act without my control. This approach is clean, sophisticated, and avoids harm to the patient. In comparison, long acting agents have a crystalline structure that stays in the joint for several weeks. These agents are known to have side effects and are bad for the long term health of joints, tendons, and the like. They are limited to three times per year in most circumstances. We do not use long acting agents, nor have we seen these side effects with extensive use of the short acting agents over 35 years.

The term steroid has been used in the national news for some time. The steroid that is discussed is not the medical type at all, which is similar to the steroids that our bodies need and produce on a daily basis. The steroids that athletes use and that have become so notorious are so-called anabolic steroids, which are derived from animal testosterone. These are developed to add protein to muscles. The problems caused by these types of drugs are not seen in the medical types. The worst that can happen to an individual who gets an injection with a short acting steroid is that there may be an increase in blood sugar if you are a diabetic, otherwise, no effects. Prolonged intake of steroid by mouth can have more side effects, and this should be followed closely by your doctor.

Non-steroidals (NSAIDs) like aspirin, naprosyn, Alleve, and Vioxx are helpful drugs for musculoskeletal injuries. It should be remembered though that for any of these medications to be effective there must be a blood supply to the injured area. Muscle tissue has a very good blood supply but ligament, joint capsule, and tendon does not. These agents are helpful, but they are not miraculous.

Narcotic use has increased again in recent years with the advent of newer medications that last for longer time periods or come as a sucker or sticker instead of a pill. Opioids can be helpful after surgery and when dealing with cancer pain for example. Narcotics may offer relief, but they only cover up pain and do not affect the inflammatory process. It was said years ago that people with pain do not get addicted to narcotics, and that they can easily come off these medications once the pain has been treated. I couldn't disagree more. I have seen people controlled by these drugs, doctor shopping for their next refill, living a life around a pill. People call my office on a daily basis, stating they have pain and they want to get off the medications. When they learn they will not be given narcotics but their pain will be treated in other ways, they do not show for their appointment. It is a sad and growing problem that has been legitimized in this country.

Other agents commonly used include muscle relaxers and anti-spasticity medications in attempts to stop painful muscle spasms. I do not espouse the use of these medications because I do not feel that the muscle is the root cause of any kind of pain beyond the first few days after injury. Anti-spasticity medications do relax muscles, but this is for the spasticity phenomenon, which follows stroke and other brain and spinal cord nerve loss. Muscle relaxers are known to inhibit the central nervous system rather than relaxing muscles.

Physicians have been prescribing anti-depressants for patients in attempts to improve their mood if they have not been successful with treating their pain. Some of these medications are particularly sedating and have been used to establish good "sleep/wake cycles". A good night's rest always makes one feel somewhat better, so these types of medications are occasionally useful. However we feel that a different approach to pain treatment, emphasizing mobility rather than strength, lessens the need for these types of medications. What may help people the most is the realization that there are new concepts for treating their problems, and they do not have to accept their pain, and they can live better in the future.

Anti-seizure medications are being used with increased frequency as doctors try to lessen the "pain signal" by blocking the nerves ability to make the impulse. In the medical literature there appears a series of articles that seems to support the fact that the nerve tissue turns on itself, causing pain by itself. My read on this problem is that the cause of the pain in the first place has not been treated. The nerves are only doing their job in this situation—the answer is to stop the process that is making the nerves fire. The pain syndrome in these articles has not been treated adequately and keeps sending a sensory response to the brain, which reportedly may cause changes. I have my doubts on hearing these experts if the changes actually appear. Those teaching and writing the articles are laboratory-types of people, who do not have a clinical practice and therefore are not aware of the many causes of pain syndromes. To be able to diagnose pain syndromes requires a different discipline, a clinical physiology oriented physician to diagnose and treat these painful problems. There is no pain source that cannot be treated in my humble opinion. So to the reader, do not accept the above scenario of neuropathic pain. I would not accept it for myself and you should not either. These medications do not affect this underlying process; therefore these drugs are not prescribed for my patients.

Chapter 22
The Political-Legal-Healthcare Tangle

The health care debate has increased lately with physician malpractice insurance and increasing health care costs raising the problem to crisis levels in some areas. It is well known that West Virginia now has no neurosurgeons, so anyone with a head injury or acute spinal cord injury had better hope they are near the state border when the injury occurred so proper care can be received quickly. The rising costs of liability insurance are only part of the healthcare mess. In this chapter I will explain to you the healthcare business from the physician's perspective. I will point out the problems with liability insurance and healthcare insurers which are slowly ruining the best health care system in the world. The problems lie in politics and laws and profit margins, with the unfortunate sick in the middle of it all.

The most notorious problem now, referenced often in the news, is the problem with physician liability insurance—malpractice insurance premiums rising too much, too fast, forcing physicians to retire or move. I hear other physicians complain almost every day regarding this issue. Now the most obvious, and most superficial, reason would be too many lawsuits. I will not downplay this because it is true in its own right—this country has become litigious. It seems no one accepts personal responsibility for their own actions. The smoker who sues the tobacco company is a prime example of this.

However the medical lawsuit it is more complex than a simple personal injury suit. The medical lawsuit must show that the physician let a Dereliction of Duty lead Directly to Damage, or the 4-Ds. The 4-Ds must be corroborated by another physician. This physician, the "head hunter" as known in medical parlance, is actually what is behind these outrageous cases. There are some physicians who will testify that any care, no matter how prudent, was ill-advised, reckless, harmful, and wrong. These physicians will testify because they are paid well. If the plaintiff does not have a physician who will testify, or "head hunt", as an expert witness, then there is no case. No case, no victory, no payout for the insurer, no increased premium for the physician, and most importantly available healthcare providers for the people. It seems simple, but only lately have the states caught on and made sure the "head hunter" actually had the expertise and qualifications to testify in a case. Often the "head hunter" will not know all the facts regarding a case and will only be allowed to review the notes. The plaintiff's attorney will not provide all of the information to the doctor, and he will offer an opinion based on a scarcity of data. If other information is known which would affect the case, the "head hunter" should be told. All the facts of the case must be exposed to the so-called expert before the trial can be done. I believe that the so called expert should talk to the physician being sued to know what was done and why, at least to know the facts. This eliminates the "Gotcha" legal case. There are two human beings in these cases, the plaintiff and the doctor. Until now the doctor is treated as an object with money and not as a professional with patient safety in his mind. Without the head hunter, there is no case.

There are medical mistakes made and I will not deny this. People often suffer for these mistakes. These people deserve compensation for their *losses*, which is the most important idea here. When a jury hears a case, they should compensate an individual for what they would have been able to do, earn, or make had there been no medical error. If an individual was making X dollars a year and was not ready to retire for 10 years, then the losses are 10X. It is that simple. Punitive damages should be the lesser of the consideration. I assure you that the physician feels the punitive damage on a daily basis. It will haunt him or her on a daily basis and there is no escape from it. Unfortunately these punitive damages can be huge dollar amounts, well beyond what the person would have been able to make. Can you put a value on "suffering"?—A hundred dollars? A billion dollars? What is the answer? What is fair? It's a difficult question to answer. Punitive damages are assessed to make sure that the mistake will not occur again. What if it never occurred in the past and the treatment was indicated?

Large jury awards force the insurer to raise insurance premiums for physicians, no matter how good they are. This cannot be denied. I hope that the people, the jurors, soon realize that they are actually the ones who lose, when they need medical care and Oh no! there is no physician for them, because the physicians couldn't afford the insurance premium. It should be known that California instituted legal reform in the 1970s for "pain and suffering" compensation with judgment caps and they have no healthcare crisis from liability insurance today. West Virginia I am told has no neurosurgeons in the state.

I think a bigger problem for physicians exists but the people do not know about it. Our biggest problem is the health insurance company, the company entrusted to assume the burden for its enrollees. This has not gotten the attention of the media yet, but I believe it will eventually. Ideally, the insurer is there to manage money. It offers health care insurance to the masses, whose monthly premiums cover the health care costs of the few who need it at the time, plus some extra for profit. One as naive as I would think that the insurance company is like a protector to me in my endeavor to have medical insurance to take care of my health. After all, I do pay the premium each month, and it is not cheap. My idea was that the insurance company would pay my physician for services that they agreed to in price and scope and I would have a better life.

The insurance company ideally should not be involved in the practice of medicine, because they are not equipped to do so, that is, the patient does not appear for examination at the insurance company offices. Therefore, the responsibility for treatment of the client must reside in the physician's office.

The insurance company will manage money—that is their job, to make sure that the premium that you pay will generate a sum of money to pay for your claim when you make one. This is done by the office staff and others at the insurance company and should be seamless for you. The above works well when each segment does their own job. What happens, when some segment of the system gets greedy?

The company will make money by limiting your access to care. Limit the physicians you can go to and they limit the money paid out. Limit the number of physicians that you can go to, and make sure that the care is not too good where the insurers tell you that they will pay for services, and limit the money paid out. The idea is that if you can't be seen by the doctor, then the insurer isn't paying money out. If the enrollee doesn't go to the doctor, then that is the way to save money. Who suffers from this business acumen?—the enrollee, the *common person*. It is shameful, yet neither the people nor the politicians have caught on yet. Hopefully they will.

How does an insurance company limit access to care? A process called *deselection*. Insurers will "include" a few physicians in their plans and "exclude" others. This is known as the "out of network" provider that is well known to everyone. The insurer will allow only so many doctors in their plan for a certain field. They must assume all physicians are equal in ability, even though it is obvious that this is not true. Any physician seeking to contract with an insurer has the risk that the insurer will state they have enough providers and is out of luck. Often state laws let the insurer do this because the law lets the insurer determine what is needed for its enrollees. I believe that this is a conflict of interest. How can the state legislature let an insurance company, which wants to make a profit, determine the people's standard of care without oversight? It is clear that the state does not offer a standard or enforce a standard because some insurers will accept physicians in their network while others do not, even though the declining insurer will have a similar share of the market. How can some insurers accept all providers and some decline them? What do the decliners use for criteria? They will not say when asked, and instead hide behind the state law. These are human lives after all, but the bottom line, what is shown to the shareholders, is more important.

I have been a victim of this by a local heath care insurer. I was told that the number of providers meets the needs of the people. I fought this for over a year, and talked to a senior vice-president of the company, who was not a physician. I was told that the market is "mature" and that the services need to be limited to "keep the costs down" and for "quality standards." This argument can be absolutely destroyed and relegated to meaningless excusatory words with little effort. The manager I spoke to thought that if there were more physicians allowed to see their enrollees the costs would rise. In other words if a service is available, then it will be used. What happens to those patients that need the service? What are the quality standards? Why are they not published by the insurance company? What happens if you do not like the designated PPO doctor? What can you do if the results of treatment take too long and you lose your job? No, the concept of the PPO is flawed, irretrievably.

The first rebuttal point I can make is that these are human lives and money is not the issue. The second point I can make is that costs *decrease* with competition, not increase. I cannot think of an instance where costs increase with competition. The marketplace will handle those practitioners that cannot handle the load any longer. They will continue to do good things for people, but more people will go to more capable providers. Thirdly, no matter how many physicians are included, the cost of treating a patient will be the same at each provider. The insurers won't pay more than they said they would—it's in the contract. If you still have your problem after the fees are paid, too bad. If an enrollee has a shoulder pain, the examination in one office will pay the same amount in another office. Why won't the insurer pay in one office when they will in another? The insurer pays the same in each case because it is in the contract—a shoulder exam costs the same amount no matter where it is performed. The way for the insurer to save money is to have accurate, rapid care at low, livable prices. The patients should decide where they want to go for their care and let the marketplace decide the cost which will be lower. The fourth point is that no insurance company has ever asked for outcome studies, or cost data, or other evidence of quality. How do they know anything about quality? The contract that physicians get with insurers mentions *nothing* about maintaining adequate standards, just ensuring that the physician provides the notes and the information so that the insurer knows what to pay. The insurer wants to make sure that the physician has liability coverage sometimes, but beyond that the insurance company does not seem to care about the quality of the care provided, just that they are provided with the office notes so that they know what to pay. The points in their deselection argument are pure fiction, intended to intimidate any challenge to their decision. I assure you that the overall bottom line drives the decisions in these cases, not the condition of the patient.

How does the insurance company get away with this? There are two pillars of support. One support is a state law that gives the insurer all the power to determine what its enrollees needs are and terminate any physician contract if this need is exceeded without explanation. This is important because by limiting the care from certain individuals, this now becomes the defacto standard of care and will be lower. The other support is to appoint physicians onto a panel that will give the company a recommendation that they are looking for, so that they can trim their provider lists. They do not ask the ones knowledgeable about the problem, however. They only do it in the dark of night so no one can see the results of the panel. Deselection off the panel without explanation is beneficial to the company and detrimental to the paying public and does help the bottom line of the favored physicians. The other reason for this statement is that the more you offer a service, the less the company will pay for it. In essence the insurers do not want the availability because they think this means people will use it, which means there will be less profits. To bring down prices, you have many suppliers of services, and then to negotiate the fees down to manageable levels. This obvious chore is not done. The in-group of physicians does, however, make a killing. By limiting the access to care for the paying public, most of the fee money goes to selected doctors regardless of their outcomes or abilities. Having politicians in the pocket of the insurance company helps the companies get away with it.

The most important aspect of the above is not the financial loss to those physicians that are deselected. It is the irrecoverable damage to their reputations in the minds of the public and the uninformed physicians. The public will assume that the insurance company is operating on their behalf and that there is a deselection for some reason. The state medical licenses and board certifications are not given without proof of expertise by these physicians. The insurance company will destroy someone's reputation to save a few dollars for themselves. Politicians do not seem to care that the standards they set by law are completely disregarded by the insurers. You can be a world-class physician with the most skill and knowledge, but without a good reputation you cannot use those skills. The public loses again. Conversely, the physicians selected are now promoted as the experts.

The physician and the patients are squeezed between a mandate for liability insurance and the insurance provider's challenges to fair reimbursement practices. Hospitals and insurance companies demand to see that the physician they contact with has liability insurance. If the insurer does not reimburse, then the provider cannot pay for the ever increasing liability insurance, and the provider cannot practice medicine. The physician has problems contracting with insurers and then cannot earn enough for the liability premium payment. Combine the two and the physician squeeze is on. Make no mistake that the only losers are the people.

Take away idea: We as consumers of health resources need access to any physician of our choice, any physician who can help us. The insurance representative cannot substitute for good care. He can only interfere with good physicians. I will not enroll in a plan for myself that limits my ability to seek out the doctor of my choice, not the insurance company choice. I am also not going to be sent to a friend of the doctor instead of the very best caliber of physician that is available. So, if a PPO is offered to you, walk away. This is especially true in the Medicare HMO. I have not been impressed with the care of the elderly in these plans. Often, patients want better care, but are in a financial bind because of the limitations put on them arbitrarily by the plan. Do the seniors need the best medical care available? Why are they treated as second class people? They have earned the right to free access of the medical establishment out there.

In my county, Anthem, or Blue Cross, limited access to care by only naming two full time physical medicine specialists, and naming many part time specialists who have their main offices in other cities around the area. The ones selected have as their main treatment regimen a stable of physical therapists, offering water therapy and exercises. The usual approach is to order many sessions of physical therapy, and to make the main provider of services the physical therapist, with the usual order of evaluate and treat. This is not good Physical Medicine and Rehabilitation that I am accustomed to in my practice, where I am the only one responsible for the care of that patient. Anthem encourages this approach. There are 49 physical medicine specialists in Columbus, Ohio, one for every 36,000 people, while in Mahoning County there are only 2 for 250,000 people. This same company eliminated 3 ophthalmologists in favor of one group. Is the care better? No one knows the outcome studies to make this assessment. If the insurance company wants to reduce costs, then why not have a round table discussion among the specialists in one field or another to discuss their findings and results so that the care will increase for the enrollees of the plan. There is no power in this approach for the insurance company, but it is good management.

Chapter 23
Physical Therapy Treatments for
Pain : What and Why

I am sure that most everyone is familiar with Physical Therapy, which is commonly used as the first-step for treating neck and back pains and other such injuries. Other chapters have touched upon physical therapy treatments, but there are many exercises and modalities that are available to you which should be clearly explained. Some are based in good science and are used in my practice, and I have discarded others. Before beginning this chapter it should be known that the physician must know all the facts about a modality so he can control the treatments. With control of the treatments, subtle changes can be made immediately to gain the best results. If the doctor writes the script for physical therapy and refers you elsewhere, he has no control over the treatment. If the doctor has no control, he or she cannot know what works and what doesn't and tailor the treatment regimen effectively. Most importantly if the doctor is not directly involved he cannot see the result and figure out *why* that result occurred. I have had control of my treatments at all times, therefore I have been able to see what works for people. My involvement allowed me to figure out *why* those treatments worked and make subtle changes to the treatment regimens and modalities that others could not be able to make.

Exercises are what patients ask about the most. It has become almost a reflex response from people that if they have an injury, they think there is a strengthening exercise they should be doing to improve it. I don't know why they assume this to be true. I have seen many patients with painful shoulders with all kinds of diagnoses that were sent into an exercise therapy program. I want to stress that we do not develop a pain because we are weak. I have seen weight lifters with pain and sedentary people without and vice versa. I have seen people with neck and back pain that have been treated with arm or leg strengthening exercises, which have no relevance to the pain. What helps people in the typical exercise routine is actually the mobilization. Any strengthening activity is accompanied by motion, and the increasing mobility is what actually provides the therapy. The strength is purely a secondary issue. Acute injuries are painful, and strengthening exercises adds force and tension to structures causing more injury and more pain. Strengthening exercises are appropriate only after there is no pain, to build strength and maintain fitness. We will return to this later.

There are several exercises that we prescribe for people routinely. These exercises are mobility exercises, or stretching exercises, and they function to restore the normal range of motion or improve the mobility of a structure that is "stuck". These exercises are tailored to the person. For example, not everyone with a backache on the right side gets the same exercise. The exercise is set to mobilize the primary source of the pain, no matter if that source is on the opposite side and causing symptoms through the "swivel effect". Remember, the tailored exercise program requires the standing x-ray to show what is stuck and what is swiveling.

In the spine the mobility exercise is dictated by the facet joint. The lumbar vertebrae have a facet joint that is 90° upright and aligned at a 45° angle to the belly button, which was shown in Chapter 7. The facet allows the lumbar spine to flex and extend, and do some side-to-side bending, but no rotation. To accommodate this design, we prescribe the Forward-Flexion left or Forward-Flexion right exercise, a maneuver that was developed by the authors of this book. The FF exercise is for the facet joint pain, which is a pain with bending forward. The FF left exercise is performed by standing with the feet spread apart slightly beyond shoulder's width. The palm of the left hand is then touched to the front of the left shin. The person should be bending at about a 45° angle to the left, and this bent position is held for six seconds for each of ten repetitions. Two or three sets of repetitions should be performed per day. The FF right exercise is performed by touching the palm of the right hand to the front of the right shin. See the picture below for this exercise. The motion helps mobilize the opposite side. For example, bending forward and to the left helps mobilize the right lower back. This is a specific exercise that requires knowing how the spine is bearing weight, which we learn from the standing x-ray.

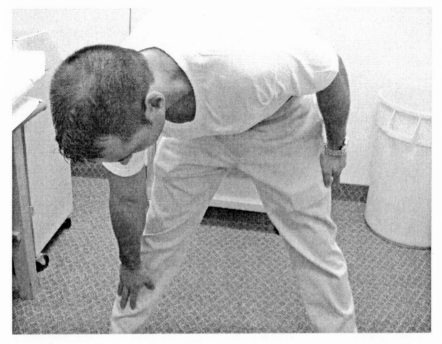

Forward-flexion right exercise. The right palm should touch the front of the right shin.

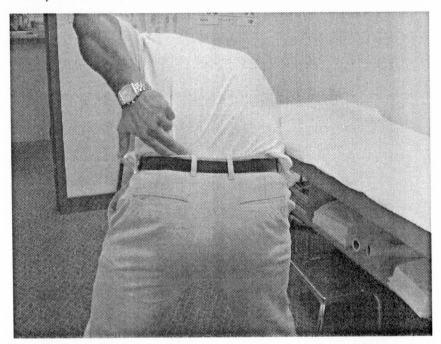

The forward-flexion right exercise mobilizes the left lower lumbar area. When doing this exercise, you should feel the stretch in the left lower back, where the model is pointing.

The thoracic spine facet joints are 60° upright and aligned 20° to the front of our bodies. This construction allows the thoracic spine to rotate. The thoracic area is kept from flexing/extending and side-to-side bending by the ribs encircling the chest. If a patient has a large curve in that part of the spine, the goal would be to straighten through a mobilization program. A curve is a result of a joint subluxation on the concave side. Please see the picture below for an example. If there is a leftward curve, then the left side needs to be mobilized. The treatment would be to rotate right, to make the left joints move. This is not muscular in nature—there is no muscle "pulling" the spine into this deformity.

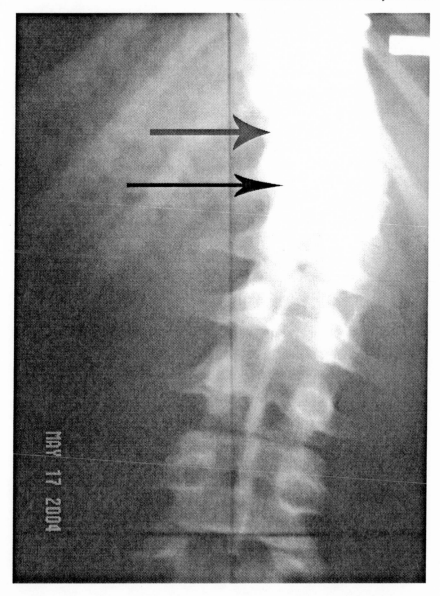

This is an x-ray of a girl with a large concave
left curve of the thoracic spine. Notice the ribs
next to the area of the spine with the greatest
curvature (arrow).

The girl had an injury causing a subluxation at the
level of the black arrow. This was treated with an
injection and her exercise was to rotate right.

Instead, this is a structural problem and the muscles have stretched to accommodate this deformity, while still being able to contract to create motion. The joint has subluxed and the component above has sunk into the one below. This dynamic exercise is aimed at actively treating this curve. A current standard for a young individual is bracing, which is a static treatment, aimed at not letting the curve progress. The person wears the brace for up to 23 hours per day, but the brace only holds the back in one place. I want to mobilize it to treat it. I do not follow the bracing approach because I believe in a dynamic treatment approach to mobilize the tight side.

The cervical spine facet joints are 45° upright and aligned roughly parallel to the front of our bodies, allowing us to nod, look to the left and right, and bend our head to the left and right. The neck is very mobile and this mobility can be injured at any level. Injuries commonly cause the neck to develop a curve, which should be straightened for the best outcome. The curve does not have to be extreme and cause a head tilt for there to be a pain. Most of the time the neck compensates above the curve to prevent a head tilt to keep the eyes level.

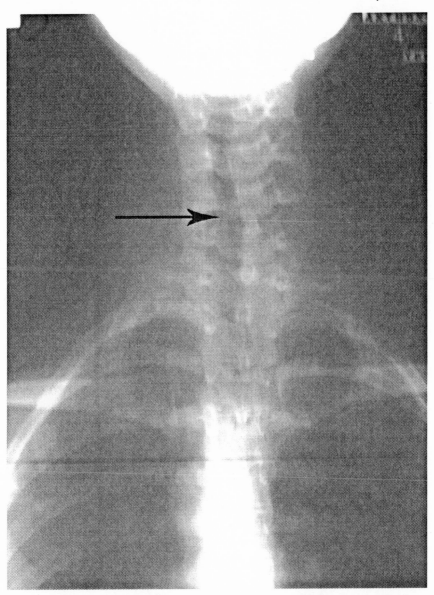

In this example of a young woman's neck, you can see
how the neck deviates to the left at the arrow.
This forces all the levels above it to be off toward
the left as well. The treatment is to mobilize the
left side by bending the neck forward and to the
right. On examination she was tender to the touch
over that left joint only.

Exercises for the neck will be a forward bend to the left or right, depending on how the neck is bearing the weight of the head. If the neck has a subluxation on the left side, like the picture above, then the exercise would be to bend forward and to the right, like the picture below. The exercise is performed by pulling the head into position for six seconds for ten repetitions. Each set is done two or three times daily.

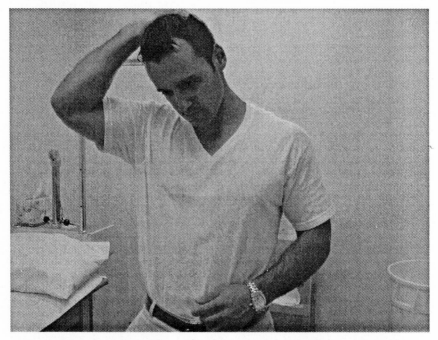

Example of a forward bend to the right, to stretch out the left neck. The head is held in this position for six seconds at a time for ten repetitions per set. Three sets should be performed daily.

I do not use strengthening exercises for neck or back pain at all, in contrast to other practitioners. The normal range of motion is what we have when we are healthy, and when we are injured we have a pain that limits this normal range. If someone moves our joint for us and we get a pain, then it means our muscle was not used and played no role in the production of that pain. In my view strength has no relevance to these structural problems, and I hope you are able to appreciate my unique viewpoint. You will not find this teaching elsewhere.

I do use strengthening exercises after treating pain when it was coming from the tendon-bone connector or muscle bone connector. This kind of pain was mentioned in Chapter 1. This cause of pain is found almost entirely in the arms or legs. The idea here is that if you exercise a muscle, the muscle bulks up like we commonly see in weight lifters. The site where the muscle attaches to the bone also gets stronger, and this is what we are trying to improve. I would never give someone the exercise when they are very painful—it just makes the symptoms worse early on. I feel the best way to treat someone is to control the inflammatory response at the injury site. This can be done by oral medication, local injection, or use of ice. This will decrease the pain for the short term and allow some comfort. After the first few days, then the goal would be to strengthen the muscle and its insertion. Initially some light exercises that do not create much tension at the injury site are ideal.

Modalities

Anyone who has been treated for pain with physical therapy in the past will be familiar with *modalities*, which are the ancillary methods used for treating pain without surgery. This includes heat and cold, ultrasound, traction, electric stimulation, TENS, magnets and others. Some methods are better than others. Some I use and some I do not because I do not like the science behind them. My goal is to familiarize you with some of these so you will be aware and knowledgeable when it comes to your treatment.

When choosing what modalities to use, the doctor or physical therapist needs to know what is causing the pain and why—there needs to be a diagnosis. Without this understanding, the modalities will not be used with a specific goal. Usually modalities provide a more broad effect for treatment, meaning the effects are not able to be focused to small, pinpoint areas but instead offer a much wider treatment area.

The first modalities I would like to mention are therapeutic heat, which is a hot pack, and therapeutic cold, which is an ice pack. The hot pack is a favorite of physical therapists. It is kept in a hot water bath to raise the temperature of the pack. When needed it is removed from the water, wrapped in towels, and applied. It provides a general warming effect of the skin and muscle and feels pretty good, like a nice, hot shower feels. However, significant pain does not originate in the skin or muscle. The hot pack does not warm deep tissue like ligament or muscle-bone connector because the skin is a good insulator. Pain originates in these deeper tissues though, and this will not be helped by a hot pack. If there is not much skin or tissue in the area, like the fingers, then a hot pack will do just fine, but I don't see many people for that kind of complaint. We do not use hot packs for patients in my office because of its superficial effect.

The ice pack is used for new injuries to prevent swelling and help with pain relief. When we have a new injury, we get the inflammatory response, which includes increased blood flow and swelling. The ice cools the skin and causes a constriction of the blood vessels which decreases the blood flow and swelling. The ice also numbs the area for pain relief. Ice is a mainstay for the treatment of acute injuries. Cold temperatures also make ligaments stiffer, analogous to a stick of butter taken from the refrigerator. It is too hard to apply to your toast until it is warmer. A basic tenet we adhere to is mobilization, which a stiff ligament cannot allow. For this reason we do not use ice for any reason beyond the acute period.

Heat improves the stretchability of ligament tissue, but as mentioned above the hot pack does not penetrate the skin well enough in most cases. Many intelligent individuals have looked into this over the years and developed the ultrasound modality treatment. Ultrasound treatment uses soundwaves, which easily penetrate the skin and fat tissue and heat the deep structures like ligaments. This is an excellent treatment choice and one of the mainstays of my practice because of its scientific basis and predictable results. You cannot have too much ultrasound because it is just a deep heat and has no detrimental effect.

Ultrasound is very commonly used by physical therapists, but not in the same manner that I use in my office. When a patient comes to my office after being treated in physical therapy, they always remark that the ultrasound treatment that I provide is different than what they experienced with the P.T. The difference is that I increase the intensity so that you will feel the heat, whereas the P.T. will say that you should not feel the heat from the ultrasound. I feel that we want to heat these deeper structures, the more the better. Raising the ultrasound intensity requires talking to the patient and watching closely however.

Some health care providers feel that ultrasound is ineffective for treating pain. I disagree because I control my ultrasound treatments and I know what to do. For example, I saw a girl who complained of pain in the neck and especially the right trapezius. The physical therapist was putting ultrasound on the trapezius area and the girl stated she did not improve from this. When I examined her, I diagnosed a C_{4-5} facet capsulitis, which refers pain to the trapezius. We treated her with ultrasound to the C_{4-5} level and she improved. The point I would like to convey to you are that modalities can be effective if the diagnosis is correct.

Another commonly used modality is traction, which is used for the neck or back. People sometimes think of this as the "rack", because it reminds them of medieval times. Traction is an excellent treatment choice, very pleasant and tolerable, which yields excellent results. People sometimes drive an hour each way to have traction treatments at my office. Traction provides a gentle stretch to the ligament structure, which is exactly what we want for our treatments. Traction for the neck can be performed lying on the back or seated. Different structures benefit from different types of traction. Traction while lying is better for the upper neck and seated traction is better for the lower levels. There are also ways to get more stretch on the left or right of the middle part of the neck or the base of the neck, depending on what areas need to be mobilized. These are techniques that I have developed on my own. In total I use eight different forms of cervical traction.

Lumbar traction can be done, though this is somewhat harder to perform. All traction requires good attachment to the body above and below the area that is to be stretched. Lumbar traction requires secure attachment to the chest and to the pelvis, which is hard to get in the typical overweight American. There are some machines that can accommodate this better than others. The most important idea to get across to you is that traction is not the best treatment for every backache. I have seen several people who have been to doctors who have done fifty or sixty or more traction treatments, without improvement. We use lumbar traction when one level is completely fixed in one area and needs to be mobilized. The result should be seen promptly or else other treatment methods should be used.

Electric stimulation is widely used by physical therapists for treating back pain. The therapist applies electrodes to the patient's skin over a painful area, and then a current is delivered to make the muscle below contract. The contraction/relaxation of the muscle is supposed to help pain in the muscle. However pain perceived from the muscle is referred from a nearby joint or the muscle-bone connector. These areas need to be mobilized. Electrical stimulation does not improve mobility, which is the key point, so I do not use it. Some people may like the way it feels while it is applied, but I think you would agree with me that all treatments should be aimed at the source for the fastest results.

The TENS unit has been around for many years, though in my experience the use of this has declined because even the physical therapists were not satisfied with the results. TENS is an acronym for Transcutaneous Electrical Nerve Stimulation, and is an offshoot of an idea that was formed in the 1960's. To put it simply, it was felt that if a nerve was stimulated at the spinal level it may block impulses from further away. There are a variety of waveforms and delivery systems but the basic concept is the same. The patient needs to experiment early on with the placement of the electrodes and delivery to get the best result. I do not use TENS because I do not believe in the underlying concept. Remember that a nerve conducts an impulse much like a telephone wire conducts a voice. The way to stop the impulse is to stop it at its source. The nerve, like the phone line, is just doing its job and transmitting an impulse. Remember a pain is a byproduct of the inflammatory response, which is itself a response to injury. Just blocking the nerve impulse does nothing for the injury, but instead lets it continue unchecked to do even more tissue damage.

Physical therapists like to use a process called iontophoresis or phonophoresis to try to get a medication into the deeper tissues, like ligament or joint capsule. Iontophoresis attempts to "drive" the medication below the skin using like charges to repel the drug, like how two similar ends of a magnet repel each other. Phonophoresis uses ultrasound to push the drug inward with a soundwave. The therapist will typically use dexamethasone, which is a specific steroid. I do not really see the point of these treatment methods because there is no way to ensure that the agent reached the structure. The drug will not be able to get deep to the ligament or muscle-bone connector. It also spreads the steroid over a broader area, which dilutes its effect and causes it to affect normal places, potentially getting into the blood stream and going all over the body. With local injection I know exactly how much steroid was put in exactly what spot. The needle prick is very small and quick and should not be the chief consideration.

Many times patients will get referred to physical therapy for water treatments or whirlpool programs. This will be a water-aerobic type program in a pool or a longer period in a hot tub. It is felt that the buoyancy of the water helps diminish some of the force on the body, allowing people to increase their activity. While this is technically accurate, I have not found this to be very useful. Any non-specific program will never give the desired outcome. It is also a time consuming and one-dimensional approach that cannot equal our other methods for pain treatment. I do not refer for a hot tub treatment either for similar reasons. The hot water from the whirlpool does not heat the source structure enough to promote more mobility.

There are other modalities which I have not listed, from lasers, to microwaves, to ultraviolet lights. Many are not being used anymore as new technology replaces the old. There likely will be other methods invented in the future which you may experience. Traction and ultrasound share the ability to soften or stretch a ligament to improve mobility. These are the only modalities that can effectively do this and these are the only modalities that I use. All other modalities are aimed at other things. I would urge you to always think of the cause and effect relationship for painful structures and ask how the treatment someone wants to give you helps that structure. I have tried to simplify most of this to provide simple and practical information. If you have any more questions, drop us a line and we will respond. (www.paintreatment.cc)

Chapter 24
24 Take Away Ideas

1. Pain treatment is part of mainstream scientific medicine. No alternative methods are needed. Alternative approaches have no scientific basis.

2. Pain is inflammatory in nature requiring anti inflammatory medication. Narcotics have no place in treatment of pain. Narcotics are not anti-inflammatory. Mild altering drugs cannot treat the real source of pain.

3. Sprain/strain is not a working diagnosis. Sciatica as a diagnosis should not be used.

4. Pain is primarily ligamentous in origin.

5. The length of time one has a pain is not a criterion for severity. Chronic pain is acute pain episodes over time.

6. MRI cannot diagnose the source of pain with certainty. MRI cannot pinpoint the source of pain. MRI is an *anatomic* study. Pain is *physiologic*.

7. Leg pain has many sources, the least of which is nerve.

8. Do not go to a physical therapist for a diagnosis or with a prescription for "Evaluate and Treat".

9. Acupuncture is only pinching the skin and cannot treat a range of motion loss. It is not scientific in its approach.

10. Electrical stimulation cannot reduce pain. Water therapy cannot treat a painful condition.

11. Bracing for pain should not be done.

12. Allopathic physicians need better education in the pain sphere.

13. Visual analog scales cannot be used to judge severity of pain.

14. Nerves do not fire off on their own causing chronic pain. There is no "Neuropathic pain."

15. 99.9% of headache is from the neck. Migraine should only mean one-sided pain.

16. Surgeons do procedures. Medical non-surgeons manage the patient.

17. Knee function is intimately related to hip function.

18. The "click" of the knee is capsular and not meniscal in origin.

19. A cool knee pain is capsular in origin.

20. Meniscal pain is primarily knee capsule in origin and should not be removed.

21. Bone-on-bone is a result of abnormal weight bearing, not of arthritis.

22. Stabilization exercises to eliminate the movements that cause pain is giving into the problem and should never be used for treatment.

23. Sitting pain noted in the leg is usually hip in origin. Sitting pain higher in the low back can be facetal in origin.

24. Low back pain with bending is easy to treat. Walking pain is always hip pain. Pain on arising from bed or a chair is hip in origin. Lumbar pain does not cause limping.

25. The recommended way to lift.
    All lifting activity should be done with the arms and legs bent. If the arms are in flexion at the elbow, then this takes the stress of lifting from the lower back. Like wise if the knees are bent the stress of lifting is taken from the lower back. When the arms are straight in lifting, the lower back will assume the burden of that weight. Bending the elbows when lifting, will cause you to bend your knees. The lumbar spine now becomes more rigid, as the base of strength for the lifting activity. I have pointed out that an injury to the low back can occur if the ligament structures are over stretched or a subluxation occurs. Holding the low back more rigid does eliminate some motion during the lifting activity. The same is true of the neck and dorsal area. The lifting thus is borne by the legs and arms.
    The so called sciatic list will occur if the lifting is done from the side with the arms straight, thus causing the low back to be unbalanced and the stress of the weight will cause a subluxation of the facet on the lifting side and a painful overstretch on the other side.
    Cervical pain can occur when the arms are straight in lifting, causing the weight of the object to be transferred to the cervical muscles and thus to be injured

26. Referred pain is a pain generated in a location away from the source.

Index

A

Acupuncture 142, 175
Ankle 102, 105, 180
Ankle sprain 105
Annulus 9
Anti-inflammatories 42
Anti-seizure medications 151
Anti-spasticity medications 151

B

Bracing 137, 138, 175

C

Capsulitis 98
Carpal tunnel syndrome 109, 110
Charcot 134
Chiropractic 43
Chondromalacia 101
Chronic pain 174
Cluster headache 46

D

Degenerative Joint Disease 16
Deselection 158
Disc 17

O

OSHA 145, 146
Osteoporosis 81, 101

P

Pain Centers. Nationwide 28, 42
Phonophoresis 172
Physical therapy 18, 43
Physiology 1, 10

R

Radiculopathy 18
Rotator cuff 61

S

Sciatica 18, 26, 174
Scoliosis 64
Sitting pain 89, 91, 176
SLAP 60
Spinal stenosis 21
Stabilization exercises 176
Strengthening 162
Subluxation 10, 21
Substance P 130

T

TENS 169, 172
Traction 171, 173
Travell 128, 129

U

Ultrasound 77, 89, 170

V

Visual analog scale 175

W

Walking pain 88, 176
Whiplash 20
Williams flexion exercises 74

Y

Yoga 142

Appendix 1

Outcome Studies

From 9/1/95 to 3/16/04 we have successfully treated:

Diagnosis	Number Days	Avg. Number of Treatment
Neck pain	3,720	4
Dorsal pain	1,450	3
Lumbar pain	3,819	3
Hip pain	1,922	4
Shoulder pain	977	3
Knee pain	1,098	5.4
Ankle pain	319	3.3
Elbow pain	420	4.0
Wrist/Hand pain	635	3.3

One hundred randomly selected Worker's Compensation patients seen between 1998-1999 were interviewed:

Average treatment days per patient: 6

92/100	returned to work to the same job
1/100	retired
1/100	works for temporary placement agency
6/100	awarded disability

94/100	require no further treatment for their pain
2/100	referred for surgery
1/100	requested surgery elsewhere
1/100	requires occasional chiropractic treatment

These statistics are nearly identical to other Worker's Compensation studies performed in 1995.

About the Author

Anthony N. Pannozzo, M.D. graduated from the Ohio State University School of Medicine in 1963, then interned at Philadelphia General Hospital. He returned to Ohio and completed residency at the Ohio State University Medical Center Department of Physical Medicine and Rehabilitation in 1967.

Dr. Pannozzo obtained board certification from the American Board of Physical Medicine and Rehabilitation in 1968 and the American Board of Electrodiagnostic Medicine in 1970. Clinical Assistant Professor at Northeastern Ohio University College of Medicine, Department of Internal Medicine.

Paul A. Pannozzo, M.D. graduated from the Northeastern Ohio Universities College of Medicine in 1999. He completed internship and residency at the Ohio State University Medical Center Department of Physical Medicine and Rehabilitation in 2003.

Dr. Pannozzo obtained board certification from the American Board of Physical Medicine and Rehabilitation in 2004.

Printed in the United States
24513LVS00004B/265-327